MacLean

NUTRITIONAL

WARFARE

Copyright 1999

A Common Sense Guide
To What's **Good** or **Bad** and Why

Medical Nutrition, Food and Health
Herbal Remedies, Food Illness, Antioxidants

by
Heather MacLean Walters, PhD

Nutritional Warfare
Copyright© August 1997 / 1999 / 2001
by Heather MacLean Walters

MCE
P.O. Box 84
Chester, NJ 07930

Cover design by Robert Alan Walters and
                    Heather MacLean Walters

Additional illustrations by Karen Duncan Bonner
and Heather MacLean Walters

Photo on back cover by Lamont Hill

Printed in the United States of America

ISBN # 0-9648913-3-6

Dedication

To my husband Rob, without whom this book, and my happiness, would not be possible.

Acknowledgments

My brother, David Cameron MacLean, Esq., has been most encouraging in all of my various endeavors. I must also give him credit for creating the title of this book.

I need to acknowledge my mother, Cynthia Maynard MacLean, who told me to write this book and who knows more about health and disease than most of the physicians that I have ever encountered. Her encouragement gave me the courage to write "not just another nutrition book". And David C. MacLean, Sr. who gave wonderful editorial guidance.

I also need to acknowledge my sister-in-law, Christa Cacciotti MacLean who was very supportive in my struggle to get this material together.

TABLE OF CONTENTS

APPENDICES

Introduction: A Call To Arms

Walking into your average supermarket these days, you are bombarded with information. Never before have so many foods been touted as "Low Fat!", "All Natural!", "Heart Healthy!", or "A Good Source of Fiber!" - in other words, good for you. Even so-called "junk food" can be made fat free, sugar free, worry free.

Modern science can engineer the food supply to make fruits and vegetables bigger, rounder, and more disease resistant. Livestock are bred to become the perfect steak or chops. And what isn't available right out of "nature" can be constructed, extruded, colored, flavored, and packaged to please even the fussiest focus group. Prime-time nutrition "specialists" would have you believe that we're on the verge of guilt-free eating, hawking diets which let you eat as much of anything you want without ever gaining weight.

Take a moment and ask yourself a simple question. Why, if all this hoopla is true, are record numbers of people afflicted with diet-related conditions like obesity, heart disease, or diabetes? Why is cancer so prevalent? How are so many new or formerly rare food-borne diseases finding their way into our communities?

Let me suggest that next time you enter your supermarket, instead of thinking of it as a carnival, you consider it what it really is - a war zone. We are all in this war, and our bodies are the battlefield. Your health, and the length and quality of your life, may ultimately depend on your ability to wage *nutritional warfare* against the forces you encounter each day.

Food is a weapon. You can be buffeted by those who do not care about your health as they use the weapon against you. Or you can take control of this weapon and change your life dramatically! The only block between you and the best use of food is knowledge. Now you can have that knowledge. All the information you need is here. Take control!

This book is designed as a practical survival guide, helping you to separate nutritional fact from hype, exaggeration and even downright misinformation. It gives you the skills necessary to evaluate your diet and make the kind of changes you need to optimize your health. While I hope you find it entertaining, it is primarily meant to be informative, and you may find it to be a slow read in places. But the results will be well worth the effort.

After you read "Nutritional Warfare" you will be prepared to do battle. And fight the good fight, for it is truly the fight of your life!

REVEILLE

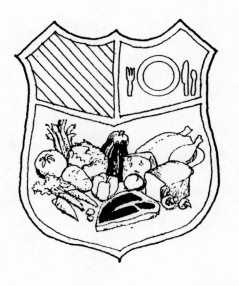

Chapter 1
WHAT IS NUTRITION?

The medical and scientific communities are beginning to realize that food is the single largest challenge facing the human immune system. In plain English, what you eat is the primary determinant of the quality and duration of your life. If that isn't a compelling enough reason for you to care about your nutrition, then you might as well put this book back on the shelf right now.

It has come as a surprise to us that food, necessary to sustain life, is a major culprit in human illness and death, directly or indirectly responsible for everything from sudden-onset food poisoning to such debilitating long-term conditions as diabetes and coronary artery disease. The good news is that food consumption is entirely within your control, unlike environmental factors and most other causes of disease. Proper nutrition and sufficient exercise are the surest tools to maximize your chances for a long and healthy life.

If you're still reading, I'll assume you care enough about yourself to be interested in how nutrition can help you achieve and maintain long-term health. The question then becomes - how?

The news is full of stories about Food X preventing Disease Y (or causing Disease Z). Some stories seem contradictory - coffee enhances thinking, but it has also been linked to colon cancer. How do you know what to believe?

I developed this book as a practical guide to deciphering the information and misinformation which faces us in the media and on the supermarket shelves every day. It won't answer every question you may have, but it will give you a background and understanding from which you can make informed choices.

As a graduate student, I was involved in a joint program in Nutrition and Food Science, under a fellowship from the U.S. Department of Agriculture. I assumed that linking these two disciplines would be a simple matter. But I soon realized that not only were these curricula vastly different, they were often at odds with each other. So, let's begin with some definitions.

Nutrition is the study of what we eat and what it does for us (and to us). Focusing on human health, it encompasses the disciplines of biology, chemistry, and physiology.

Food Science is the study of the physics and chemistry and engineering of food substances, packaging, processing and delivery of specified characteristics to the consumer. It includes the disciplines of Food Engineering, Food Biology, and Food Chemistry. It is much less concerned with health promotion and more concerned with encouraging the consumer to purchase specific products.

Nutrition is defined as the sum of the biochemical and physiological processes involved in the absorption of nutrients and the effect on growth, repair and maintenance of an organism.

Food can be defined as any substance taken into the body for physiological or psychological reasons that provides nutrition or energy.

There are several types of people that can be found in the nutritional arena. They have varying credentials with regard to nutrition and are described below.

A Nutritionist

A Nutritionist is anyone who has any knowledge or interest in nutrition, and wants to call themselves a nutritionist. There are no exacting specifications for the term, "Nutritionist". It is also used for both a person with a four-year undergraduate knowledge of nutrition (or any other subject) as well as a person with a Ph.D. in nutrition (or any other subject). It is therefore important to note exactly what credentials your nutritionist has before buying into all that he/she has to say.

A Food Scientist

A Food Scientist is anyone with a four-year undergraduate degree, Masters degree, or Ph.D. in food science. There is little distinction made here either. Even those without any degree in food science can refer to their experience alone and call themselves food scientists.

A Dietician

A dietician is a person with a two- or four-year undergraduate degree in dietetics. This person may or may not be licensed. If they are licensed, the license is the R.D. (Registered Dietician). This designation allows that the person has certain basic knowledge about nutrition and health. These individuals are limited in their knowledge for the general population, though, because they focus heavily on hospital nutrition and enteral formulas (feeding tube recipes). While vital to the hospital staff, they may be lacking in current nutritional knowledge. (For more information, see the "Who can you trust" section in Chapter 17.)

Chapter 2
WHY WE EAT WHAT WE EAT

An episode of a popular television sitcom had the main character eating at a very casual steakhouse instead of his usual trendy, healthful restaurant. It was a humorous, but traumatic experience for the delicate, refined individual which included this dialogue:

"What are those things on my potato?"
"Bacon bits."
"Oh, my God - I gave up bacon because of the nitrates!"

My response would have been: *"Don't worry, it's probably only imitation bacon-flavored textured soy grits..."*

The point is that food science has taken us very far from whole and natural foods, and closer to processed and engineered foods. **Processing** should not be confused with **Refining** or **Dismembering** food. Refining is the further purification of a desired substance or quality; dismembering is the separation of specific substances from whole foods. We process our foods at home as well as buying pre-processed foods.

Processing does not cause total loss of nutrients, only partial loss. Major losses occur when grains have bran and germ removed, alcohol is distilled, or sugar is refined. To tell how whole a food is, you can look at

Processing includes:
Freezing
Canning
Blanching
Cooking
Drying
Peeling
Mashing
Extruding

the potassium content. Potassium is found inside the cells of your food, and losses occur when the cells of a food are broken or disrupted. Ideally, we should all be eating as many whole foods as possible, To make whole food choices, ask yourself why you're eating what you're eating, how whole the food is and how much of your diet includes whole foods.

Our Food Supply

The food supply exists as **Whole (intact)** or **Partitioned** foods. Whole foods are those that come to us relatively unprocessed like fruit. Partitioned foods are those pieces of whole foods that we deem worthy of isolation, like sugar from corn or cane, oil from seeds, or fiber from oats.

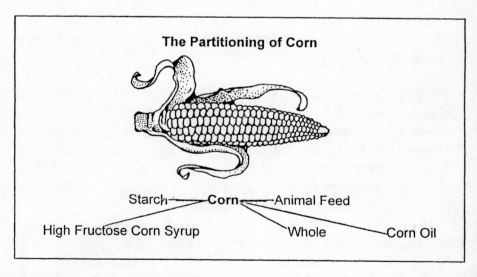

The Partitioning of Corn

Starch ————Corn———Animal Feed

High Fructose Corn Syrup   Whole   Corn Oil

Partitioned foods can be further divided into **Fabricated** foods and **Formulated** foods. An example of formulated food is Coke™ made with carbonated water, sugar and some ingredients I promised my uncle I would not reveal. Fabricated foods are those that are also known as convenience foods. They are very partitioned and removed from the original source. Margarine, Cool Whip™, and Hamburger Helper™ are a couple of examples. They can't really stand on their own as consumable, but are used to enhance other foods.

Why We Eat What We Eat

The reasons why we choose the foods that we choose are many and varied. The list below suggests a few of them, but you will undoubtedly have your own reasons as well.

Personal Preference
We all have certain foods that we like. They may or may not have nutritional value. We just like them. Our tastes are partly genetically determined, partly due to our age, and partly due to other factors including foods that we were raised to eat. Other factors include the time of day; simpler, sweeter foods are preferred in the morning (muffins / toast) and more complex are preferred later in the day (salads / casseroles).

Familiarity
While familiarity breeds contempt in certain situations, food isn't one of them. We like what we know. It's safe. Not like those icky foreign foods. Xenophobia rears its ugly head when it comes to eating out of our ethnic groups. Not with me though. I'm Scottish. Thank you, I'll have Indian, Chinese, Japanese, anything but haggis...But for most of us, old habits die hard.

Social Reasons
"Happy Birthday To You; Happy Birthday To You...I'm So Happy I'll Just Eat This Piece Of Cake With Ice Cream...Happy Birthday To You!" That's not really how the song goes, of course, but think of the times you've eaten to be friendly or sociable...How many

slices of pizza have you ingested to be part of the gang? How many times have you considered breaking your food habits just because you were worried that someone would ridicule you?

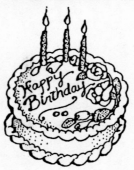

Values and Beliefs

There are certain foods, such as Kosher foods, that must be consumed at certain times of the year. Wine is offered in Christian churches every Sunday; and many denominations require the priest or minister to drink all that is left! The minister might become concerned that all that alcohol, depending upon how much is left, might do his liver in. He must drink it though because it is part of his belief system.

Availability

If it's available, you eat it. Isn't it the truth? How many times have you found yourself eating something odd in front of the television and said, "What am I doing?" It's so easy to snack on whatever is around because we're bored. Nutrition isn't even an issue here.

Temptation

It looks too good to pass up. Someone just brought over your favorite dessert and you know you shouldn't. Or you have amazing leftovers from last night's party. Who could resist? What I tell my students is to use the 80/20 rule. If 80% of the time, you're eating fruits and vegetables and only good foods, then 20% of the time you can cheat without fear of disaster.

Convenience
It was Napoleon who officially developed the first convenience foods after his encounter with Russian troops in 1812. The Russians were very clever and cut off supply lines to the French, destroying the French advance. Napoleon later vowed to always keep a supply of ready-to-eat food with his army. It wasn't long before companies like Underwood™, Borden™, Campbells™, and Birdseye™ followed with commercially-made convenience foods. Convenience foods have always been a necessity have for the thousands of men and women we send on long missions around the world.

Actually we have NASA (The National Aeronautics and Space Administration) and the armed forces (Army, Air Force, Navy, Marines, etc.) to thank for more recent convenience foods. The first TV dinners were made for Air Force pilots out on mission. B-52s were then stocked with frozen food for the troops on the ground courtesy of Swanson™.

NASA has always needed food that did not perish in unusual conditions, provided good nutrition to its astronauts, and could be consumed in a weightless atmosphere. Tang™, the orange breakfast drink, was one of the many foods developed for space exploration. I think it was our interest in space exploration and new frontiers that led us to embrace these new convenience foods so quickly. Desert Storm led to the creation of foods that met even more stringent criteria; including the ability to survive for months in excessive heat.

When we've had a long day, we sometimes say, "I'm too rushed too cook, I'll just eat this." I can't count the number of times that I've been too busy for major food preparation and have opted for a convenience food. Using convenience or pre-prepared foods too often can have negative ramifications on your diet, like excess sodium and fat. Planning ahead to feed your family properly, by freezing your prepared casseroles or dishes, is often just as convenient; and addresses the next reason for food choice, economy.

Economy
"The least expensive product, that's what I'll buy." When we're on a budget or need to conserve our resources, we tend to gravitate towards the inexpensive or generic version of a food. This allows us to have the type of food we desire and still stick to our budget. In the "Nutritional Tips For A Cancer-Free Life", I suggest that this may be the wrong way to go. If you want ice cream and are on a budget, you are better off saving the calories and buying fruit or buying the small version of the expensive, well-known brand. Well-known brands are more likely to use standard practices of cleanliness and preparation; and they have toll-free numbers you can call if there is a problem. To economize, buy more fruits and vegetables than prepared foods. You'll be surprised at the savings.

Reward or Consolation
Food, especially fatty food, is texturally comforting and we often seek such foods when we're feeling low. Lost your job? Dumped by your boyfriend or girlfriend? It's time for the Haagen-dazs™, the Oreos™, the huge bag of chips. Nearly everyone seeks consolation in food sometime or another. This is perfectly fine, if you only do it on a rare occasion. If, however, you're forever drowning your troubles in food, you need to talk to someone or

find some sort of activity to substitute for the quick gratification of food.

Nutritional Value

You perceive a food to be good for you. We all listen to the news on television, read the paper, ask our neighbors and friends advice, and then make choices about nutrition from these sources. In many cases, this is O.K. But in some cases, what someone has told us is "just what you need" may harm us. In a later section there is a list of people you can trust to give you fairly sound nutritional advice. These are the people you should count on when looking for a nutritional solution.

RECONNAISANCE

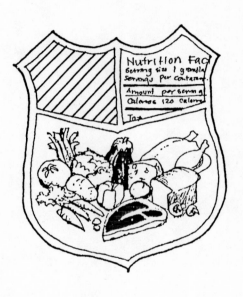

Chapter 3
READING LABELS

The most convenient source of nutritional information for most packaged foods is the "Nutrition Facts" label. Reading and interpreting the information on the label is an important part of your nutritional reconnaissance. This chapter provides some guidelines for getting the most out of these labels. You may want to reread this chapter after gaining more of an understanding of fats, carbohydrates, proteins, vitamins and minerals.

What's On Our Current Nutrition Labels?

The following pieces of information were required to be on most nutrition labels by 1993:

Required Listed Nutrients

Calories
Calories from fat
Total fat (grams)
Saturated fat (grams)
Cholesterol (milligrams)
Total carbohydrates (grams)
Complex carbohydrates (grams)
Sugars (grams)
Dietary fiber (grams)
Protein (grams)
Sodium (milligrams)
Vitamin A (% of Daily Value)
Vitamin C (% of Daily Value)
Calcium (% of Daily Value)
Iron (% of Daily Value)

This labeling standard was imposed by the U.S. Food and Drug Administration (FDA) and the Food Safety and Inspection Service (FSIS). What does this mean to you, the consumer? It depends. It is nice to know the hard facts like how many grams of protein you are ingesting, but there are "soft" facts as well. I find it to be of no use to know the "% of Daily Value" that a serving of a food supplies. What does that mean? Why should I care?

"% Daily Value" means "the percentage of nutrient in a particular food that is necessary in the diet of a 150 pound man who eats 2500-3000 calories of prescribed amounts of nutrients per day". Good luck deciphering that if you are not a 150 pound man or you eat irregular amounts of everything.

The bottom line is that these "% Daily Value" labelling regulations do not help you at all. As an individual with different caloric intake, lifestyle and weight, you need "...just-the-facts-ma'am." But just as a camel is a horse designed by a committee, some of these FDA/FSIS regulations come out less than perfect. And you are provided with less information than you need and more fluff than you want. Other measuring systems are discussed in the table at the end of this chapter, and these are also of limited practical value. To obtain meaningful information on your nutritional intake, use the guidelines in this book for total nutrient intake, rather than relying on percentages.

There are also voluntary disclosures that food processors and manufacturers can make, like the amount of other minerals and vitamins. These, of course, would only be listed if it were to the manufacturer's benefit. Labeling is expensive and often fought at every turn by food companies. Small companies or those with small packaging (less than 12 square inches) are exempt from many of the labeling requirements.

Deciphering Label Contents

On the following page is a sample label from a container of organic milk I recently purchased. Let's go over it in detail, examining the contents and their importance in your diet analysis.

Organic Skim Milk

Ingredients
First look at the ingredients to find out what is actually present in the food. In this first case, the only ingredients are skim milk, Vitamin A and Vitamin D-3. These vitamins are the fat- soluble vitamins, and you might figure that consuming them without fat present might hinder their absorption. You'd be both right and wrong. Yes, you need to eat food that contains fat in order for good absorption of fat soluble vitamins, but skim milk has fat! That's right, it has 1/2% fat content.

Serving Size
It is very important to determine the amount of fat, protein, calories and other things that you get in one serving. Next, it is important to determine whether the manufacturer of the food is trying to call something a "serving" that is less than that which you'd actually consume. In this case, one cup or 8 ounces of milk is about what the average person would consume in one sitting, so the serving size is about right.

Watch for labels with unrealistically small serving sizes. This is a widely used trick that allows manufacturers to claim lower fat, calories, or just about anything else per serving. The label on a bag of vending machine potato chips may look low-fat, until you notice that that little bag is actually supposed to be 2 (or more) "servings".

Keep Refrigerated
Pasteurized Homogenized
Vitamin A & D   Grade A
Organic Skim Milk

Nutrition Facts

Serving Size 1 cup (236 mL)
Servings Per Container 8

Amount Per Serving

Calories	80
Calories from Fat	0

	% Daily Value
Total Fat 0g	0%
Saturated Fat 0g	0%
Cholesterol less than 5mg	1%
Sodium 130mg	5%
Total Carbohydrate 12g	4%
Dietary Fiber 0g	0%
Sugars 12g	
Protein 8g	16%

Vitamin A 10% • Vitamin C 2%

Calcium 30% • Iron 0% • Vitamin D 25%

*Percent Daily Values are based on a 2,000 calorie diet. Your daily values may be higher or lower depending on your caloric needs:

	Calories	2,000	2,500
Total Fat	Less than	65g	80g
Sat Fat	Less than	20g	25g
Cholesterol	Less than	300mg	300mg
Sodium	Less than	2,400mg	2,400mg
Total Carbohydrate		300g	375g
Dietary Fiber		25g	30g

Calories per gram:
Fat 9 • Carbohydrates 4 • Protein 4

INGREDIENTS:
CERTIFIED* ORGANIC
SKIM MILK, 2000 I.U. OF
VITAMIN A PALMITATE
AND 400 I.U. OF VITAMIN
D_3 ADDED PER QUART.

***CERTIFIED ORGANIC
BY**

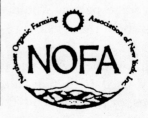

**PLEASE FLATTEN
CONTAINER
PRIOR TO
DISPOSAL TO
SAVE LANDFILL
SPACE**

Calories (per serving)

A calorie is a measure of the energy provided by a food. Caloric value is measured scientifically by burning the food and measuring the heat energy produced. Our bodies "burn" calories in much the same way, though not all calories are equal in terms of how easily they can be converted to energy.

Total calorie intake is a simple and convenient nutritional measure. You should figure out what you're eating by estimation (1 serving, or 5 servings!) and keep track of your caloric intake. Try it for 3 days using the 3-day diet analysis in the appendix. Do not be tricked by the serving size on the package, as described earlier. Make your own estimates.

How many calories should you consume daily? The answer is - it is different for every individual. Your ideal caloric intake will vary depending on your age, gender, size, and activity level. These factors influence your energy output. And of course, you're trying to strike a balance between input and output.

In general, adult women have a baseline resting energy expenditure (REE) of 1300 - 1400 calories per day; for men, this figure is between 1600 and 1800 calories per day. To account for our daily activity, total energy allowance is figured by multiplying the REE by some value, typically around 1.6 - 1.7. This implies that caloric intake should be 2000 to 2200 calories for women and 2500 to 3000 calories for men. Having said this, I say again: everyone is different, and you'll need to experiment to find the intake level that's right for you.

Ultimately, calorie counting alone is of limited utility, and what you eat is every bit as important as how many calories that food contains. Just remember the one inescapable fact: if you take in more calories than you expend, you will store and accumulate this energy - and gain weight.

Calories from Fat (per serving)
A gram of fat has 9 calories, while a gram of protein or carbohydrate has only 4. This is why most high-fat foods are also high in calories. A useful rule of thumb is that you should restrict your calories from fat to 30% of your total calories.

While not as important as total calories or total grams of fat consumed, this can give you an indication as to whether you are close to the 30%-calories-from-fat goal. It won't help you to look at this number unless you do the math below. And it won't help you to know the percentage unless you do the math for all the foods you eat and then average them. I know this is a lot of math, but it's worth trying at least once, over a 3- or 6-day period.

Step 1 - For Each Food:

Calories from Fat   =   Percentage of calories from fat
  Total Calories

Step 2 - For All Foods Eaten In A Day:

Food 1	Calories from fat	Total calories
Food 2	Calories from fat	Total calories
Food 3	Calories from fat	Total calories
Food 4	Calories from fat	Total calories
Food 5	Calories from fat	Total calories
Food 6	Calories from fat	Total calories
All Foods:	Calories from fat	Total calories

Calories from fat (all foods)   =   Total Percent Fat For One Day
Total calories (all foods)

Step 3 - Total Percent Fat In Diet: Add up all your "Total Percent Fat For One Day" figures and divide by the total number of days that you test yourself. This will give you an indication of the percentage of your diet that is fat. This can be done for any single nutrient, like protein or carbohydrates. It is only an approximation, not an accurate measure. Adding grams of fat together is an accurate measure, provided you know the tricks (see "Tricks of The Trade", Chapter 25).

Total Fat (per serving)
This is a very important number when looking at how to adjust your diet for better health. Total fat consumption should not exceed 30 grams per day, but you should also never go less than 10 grams per day or serious problems could develop. Much easier than calculating percentage, it gives you a raw, easy-to-interpret number that you can work with. In our example label, the total fat is listed as 0 grams. In this case there is so little fat it was correctly deemed unimportant to mention. But while "0" grams is not exactly true, many companies also follow the deceptive industry standard (see Tricks of the Trade).

Saturated/Monounsaturated/Polyunsaturated Fat (per serving)
OK, now you know exactly what percentage of fat you eat per day and exactly how many grams on average. But what kind of fat is it? And how important is that difference? We'll discuss these questions in depth in Chapter 6.

Current research suggests that it is better to eat mostly monounsaturated fat because it is less likely to cause hardening of the arteries, heart problems or cancer. Monounsaturated fats are better for the phospholipid bilayer of your cells.

Saturated fat can clog arteries or help propel cancer along. But saturated fat is much more difficult to oxidize and may be better than polyunsaturates if cancer is your only concern.

Switching to polyunsaturates may be the easiest fix for those with heart problems who eat a diet rich in saturated fat. But polyunsaturates can easily be oxidized, setting up a pre-cancerous situation. This oxidation also takes place in your arteries and polyunsaturates can help precipitate some plaque problems.

I have often said, with great regret, that my wonderful Grandpa Maynard died of cream pie. And I believe it to be true, for he developed a wild and rampant version of cancer that affected lung, prostate, and other organs in his body. It was not exactly determined where the cancer began. But I know that it began when he started eating banana cream, pecan and other sorts of pies filled with polyunsaturated fatty acids for breakfast, lunch and dinner.

It also serves as a good example of what you can and cannot do for people. I tried very hard to help him adjust his diet, bringing him fruit and vitamins and suggesting that we not go to his favorite pie restaurant all the time, but he wouldn't listen. Sure he loved me, but what did a young college kid know? You should try and gently give sound nutritional advice to your friends and relatives, but know when to back off or give up. It is only really you that you can work on.

I asked a renowned lipid expert from Rutgers University what kind of substance she put on her toast in the morning. Her reply was telling. "Nothing", she said. "Not even jam?", I asked. "No, it raises your triglycerides." I think she was offering good advice. What she was telling us was to control our lipid intake by not slathering all of our food willy-nilly with butter, margarine or jam.

Cholesterol (per serving)

<u>Forget about it</u>. I regularly tell my students to forget about the cholesterol content of food. It is unimportant. What is important, however, is the total fat content, saturated fat content, and consumption of vegetables and fruits in your diet. These three things if properly ingested will affect your own cholesterol count the most.

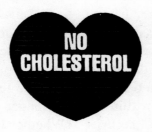

Cholesterol is only found in animals. There is an annoying tactic that vegetable and fruit producers use to con the public. "Cholesterol Free" labels and signs have appeared with just about every form of produce whose producers feel that they will gain an advantage over some other vegetable or fruit producer. After all, some of us have to worry about our cholesterol count and the foods we eat. So the produce people prey on our fears and make us feel compelled to buy a particular vegetable. Once and for all, I scream:

FRUITS AND VEGETABLES HAVE <u>NO CHOLESTEROL</u>!!!
They <u>never</u> have had any cholesterol!

As animals, we make our own cholesterol every day (about 11 mg per deciliter of blood)! But we can lower our intake of saturated fat and lower our ability to produce large amounts of cholesterol. This lowered intake of saturated fat works if there is no genetic predisposition to higher cholesterol production, no post-menopausal spike in cholesterol, no surge in production that can come in later life and if you are sure of your cholesterol number.

To be sure of your cholesterol number you should have it taken at least three times. It changes after a meal, when you've been upset, in the morning versus the afternoon, whether you have been eating well weeks before they ask you to fast the night prior to the test. The reason you're asked to fast is to get the lowest possible reading and use those numbers to diagnose any problems. But a false low could be dangerous for someone who regularly eats heavily fatty meals and then fasts for the test. This fasting might produce a number within normal ranges and give doctor and patient a false sense of security. (Whether your cholesterol is high or not, if you eat a lot of fat or meat, stop now and save your life!)

Lowering saturated fat works, because all of the cholesterol we ingest is found along with the largest portion of saturated fat that we can find--in the flesh of dead animals! Put down the bacon, ease off the lobster, lower shrimp intake, use ersatz hamburger and, BINGO! Lower cholesterol!!!

Now, note that vegetable oils, nut butters and fruits like avocado should also be eaten in smaller amounts if your cholesterol is dangerously high. These provide lots of fat we don't need, while also providing good nutrition. Use them in moderation.

Total Carbohydrate (per serving)
This number gives you an indication of the carbohydrates you ingest per serving, but is not helpful when it comes to looking at your health status in reference to carbohydrates, because the kind of carbohydrates you eat is more important than the total quantity of carbohydrate. I'll have more to say about carbohydrates in Chapter 8.

Complex Carbohydrates (per serving)

These are the most important kind of carbohydrate you ingest. The more of them you eat, the healthier you will be. Complex carbohydrates include those carbohydrates more commonly referred to as "Fiber". For a discussion of the different types of fiber, see the Carbohydrates chapter. This number should be higher than the sugars in your diet.

Sugars / Simple Carbohydrates (per serving)

Sugars are a source of energy and we need them in order to live, but too much refined sugar (including all dark brown, light brown, turbinado, raw and white varieties) is not good for us. It has been suggested that too much simple sugar predisposes us to diabetes, cancer and obesity. And now maybe the *Body Browning Reaction* too! (See the "Aging" section in Chapter 16.)

Dietary Fiber (per serving)

This number along with sugars is additive and should reflect total carbohydrates. Dietary Fiber takes two basic forms, soluble and insoluble. The type of food is indicative of the type of fiber contained therein. Oats, for example, contain soluble fiber which gets into your bloodstream and is good for your heart; raisin bran contains insoluble fiber which is good for your digestive system. You need both kinds of fiber in a healthy diet.

Protein (per serving)

It is necessary to know the number of grams of protein in each of the foods you consume. This gives you an idea whether you are near the 40 - 50 grams deemed necessary by current nutritional standards. Add the number of grams of protein in all of your foods and see if you are getting enough daily protein. More information on protein is provided in Chapter 7.

If all of the protein you ingest is taken along with insoluble fiber, such as that found in bran cereal, you should adjust the grams of protein. Protein taken along with great amounts of insoluble fiber is poorly absorbed, so take the number of grams and divide it at least in half. The halved number is a high estimate of the actual number of grams of protein that were available to you. You should eat your protein separately from your fiber if you can.

Vitamins A, C, and D (per serving)
Vitamins are added to numerous products. As in the organic milk example, the vitamin value represents added vitamins, and is seldom reflective of the natural vitamin content of the food, unless it is a whole canned or frozen vegetable. Yes, you are getting a certain amount of these vitamins, but here, too, you must be careful to look at the fiber that is ingested with the vitamins. Vitamins are discussed in detail in Chapter 10. There is also a danger with added vitamins. In the Antioxidants section of Chapter 15, the potential dangers of such additions are explained in Secret #1.

Sodium/Calcium/Iron (per serving)
Minerals added to cereals and processed foods can be well absorbed. Once again, though, it is important to look at the type of food in which the minerals are found. Here, in the organic milk, there is a higher probability that calcium absorption will supersede that of iron, for example, because the medium is a natural calcium source and there is Vitamin D to help.

Sodium in milk is not as relevant as we'd like to think either; it is offset by a nearly perfect amount of potassium and poses little threat even to the sodium-sensitive person. The minerals are often listed as percent of daily value which, as I said before, is confusing and of little value. Chapter 11 contains an in-depth review of minerals in the diet.

RDA EXERCISE

OK, now it's your turn. Take the label of the milk you drink at home (or use our skim milk label) and list the following nutrients. They can be found on the back label of your carton or plastic jug. When you have finished filling in this chart, try the questions that follow. They will reveal a lot about how to estimate and calculate nutrient concentrations in your foods.

Nutrients Per Serving

Nutrient	Quantity		% of Daily Intake	
Fat	0 grams	___	0%	___
Protein	8 grams	___	16%	___
Carbohydrate	12 grams	___	4%	___
Vitamin A		___	10%	___
Vitamin D		___	25%	___
Vitamin C		___	2%	___
Calcium		___	30%	___
Sodium	130 mg	___	5%	___

Serving size	236 ml. (1 cup)	_____
Servings per container	8	_____
Calories per serving	80	_____

Questions

1)   **How many calories of each nutrient is found in one serving of milk?**

Example: **For Protein**
8 Grams per serving x **4 Calories** per gram
8 Grams   x   4 Calories   = 32 calories of Protein
This means that for each serving of milk, there are 32 calories of PROTEIN.

CALCULATE THESE VALUES

For Fat

Grams of fat x **9** Calories per gram

_____X_____ = _____Calories of FAT

For Carbohydrates

Grams of Carbohydrate x **4** Calories per gram

_____X_____ = _____Calories of Carbohydrate

2A) **How much of your daily Mineral requirements could you obtain if you had three glasses of this organic milk?**

Sodium per serving = 130 mg (5%)
Sodium per serving X 3   =   5% X 3   =   **15%**

Calcium per serving = 30%
Calcium per serving X 3   =   30% X 3   =   **90%**

2B) **How many minerals would you obtain from your milk? Do this for each listed mineral.**

Sodium per serving = ___ mg   =   __%
Sodium per serving X 3   =   __% X 3   =   __%

Calcium per serving = __%
Calcium per serving X 3   =   __% X 3   =   __%

3A)   How much of your daily Vitamin requirement could you obtain if you had three glasses of this organic milk?

Vitamin A per serving = 10% X   3   =   **30%**
Vitamin D per serving = 25% X   3   =   **75%**
Vitamin C per serving = 2% X   3   =   **6%**

3B)   How much of your Vitamin requirement could you get from your milk?

Vitamin A per serving = __% X   3   =   __%
Vitamin D per serving = __% X   3   =   __%
Vitamin C per serving = __% X   3   =   __%

4A)   Calculate the percentage of protein calories in one serving.

$$\frac{\text{Protein calories}}{\text{Total Calories}} \quad = \quad \frac{32}{80} \quad = 0.4 = \textbf{40\%}$$

4B)   Do the same calculations for Fat (Using a milk that <u>has</u> fat listed per serving) and for Carbohydrate.

$$\frac{\text{Fat calories}}{\text{Total calories}} \quad = \quad \underline{\quad} \quad = \underline{\quad} \quad = \underline{\quad}\%$$

$$\frac{\text{Carb. calories}}{\text{Total Calories}} \quad = \quad \underline{\quad} \quad = \underline{\quad} \quad = \underline{\quad}\%$$

Now you should be able to calculate how much of any given nutrient you get from any food. This will help with your 3- or 6-day nutritional assessment (see Appendix III), or whenever you want to evaluate a food or your diet in general.

How Much Should You Have Of Each Nutrient?

The RDA

It used to be referred to as "Recommended Daily Amount", but scientists became worried about overdoses of certain vitamins and officially changed it to "Recommended Dietary Allowance". Notice the missing component. Time! In a year, a month, a week? The answer is about 4 days. The RDA is the amount that you should have in your diet in about a 4 day period. The RDA is seldom used on labels because it is specific to different ages and sexes.

The DRV

This number covers nutrients which have no RDA, like fat, fiber and carbohydrate. This asks you to compare your dietary percentages with what are currently considered "Good" amounts, like 30% total fat or 60% carbohydrate in the diet. On every food label you will see these numbers in comparison to 2000 or 2500 caloric intake. If you eat less or more than that, these numbers are almost useless to you. The only way to estimate with these numbers is to know your exact caloric intake, divide it by the 2000 or 2500 calories on the box, and backtrack to make sure your fat intake, for example, is at the same percentage level as your calories. Too much work!

The RDI

The "Reference Daily Intake" numbers are the highest RDA for each nutrient. This was done to insure that nutrients like Vitamin B-12 and folate, and antioxidant nutrients like Vitamin E would be taken in large enough amounts to be protective. There is currently a move to change the RDI, to lower the values. Scientists see the high RDI as potentially dangerous. Vitamin manufacturers are quite concerned about their own economic fate.

The ESADDI

Known as the "Estimated Safe and Adequate Daily Dietary Intake", this is often used for nutrients without an RDA or nutrients that have not been adequately studied like Biotin, Chromium, Fluoride, etc. It is a range that your consumption of nutrients should stay within.

THE
BATTLEFIELD

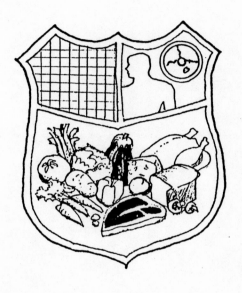

Chapter 4
WHAT'S INSIDE YOUR CELLS?

The Little Things

We will be discussing parts of your body systems, your cells, your food supply, and many other critical aspects of your nutritional life in this book. It is therefore important to tell you the story of "the little things" that help to put all of this together.

These little things are the smallest pieces we can name when describing you or your food. They are called **elements** or **atoms**. These atoms are the smallest components of your body and your food. They include the components of you, your food, and everything you see and know. If, for example, you buy a bottle of zinc supplements at the store, you will be getting the atom or the element, zinc. If you eat the zinc tablets, you will be adding the element, zinc, to your cells and bloodstream.

In the bottle, zinc will probably be attached to some other group of little things or atoms (like gluconate), so that it is absorbed more easily. In your body, the zinc will (most likely) let go of its attachment (to gluconate) from the bottle and bond or hook-up with something in your cells.

Whenever atoms or elements are stuck together, like the zinc and the gluconate, we refer to them as **molecules** or **compounds**. They can be simply two small atoms stuck together, like sodium and chlorine. When sodium and chlorine are linked, we have table salt, or sodium chlor<u>ide</u> (we change the last part in order to tell that the chlorine is hooked up with something).

These bonded, or connected, atoms can form very large groups, like fats and sugars. There are hundreds of atoms or "little things" all stuck together in fat and sugars. When we eat these larger molecules, they usually break down into useful bits with which our cells can make something else.

Your Cells

Life is chemistry. Molecules are continually being made from atoms and broken down into smaller molecules or atoms in myriad ways in living organisms. Our cells are little chemical factories that make us, the larger factory, function. Day after day they chug away making certain this enzyme goes here, that sugar is properly used, the right chemicals are excreted, etc. A microcosm of ourselves, they contain all of our genes and all of our necessary functions.

Why are cells different? It is a question I have often encountered in my teaching. It goes back to the basic set-up of life. Atoms become molecules, molecules join together to become cells (e.g. red blood cells), cells that specialize become organized into tissues (e.g. blood), tissues together become organs (e.g. the heart) and organs join one another in organ systems (e.g. the circulatory system). A liver cell is different from a skin cell, for example, in a number of ways. It has slightly different visible features than the three main types of skin cells. It has different functions, different products it produces, different turnover and reproduction times.

Whether a cell becomes a liver, skin or other specialized cell is largely determined by the turning on or off of particular genes in the first few days of our embryonic lives. This turning off or on allows certain functions to remain, certain shapes to be retained, etc. It is crucial to our existence to have this alteration of expression in the very beginning. It doesn't mean that the genes aren't the same in every one of your cells; visually they are. Some are just turned off and some are on. What we can see under the microscope doesn't tell us everything we need to know about functions, either.

What I will describe for you in this chapter is the basic cell. While liver cells and skin cells differ in functionality and external appearance, they both have the same basic components as all the cells of your dog's body, that oak tree in your yard and of your own cells. In other words, all cells are basically the same. Examples of the differences between plant and animal cells are shown on the next few pages.

The Organelles

We are animals. Our bodies are divided into organs and organ systems. Examples of organs are heart, kidney, skin, brain. Examples of organ systems are circulatory, excretory, immune, and central nervous systems. These organs work separately, in coordination within their respective systems, and in concert with the other systems in a healthy body.

Your cells are very much the same, only on a smaller scale. They too have organs, only they are so small we have to call them "organelles". These organelles also must work together inside your cells to digest your food, to coordinate enzyme and hormone reactions and release, and many other vital functions.

The Order Of The Chemistry Of Life
(From Smallest to Largest)

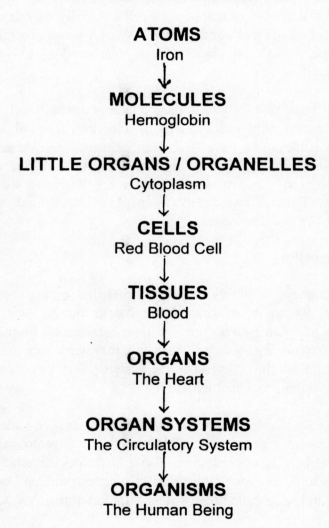

ATOMS
Iron
↓

MOLECULES
Hemoglobin
↓

LITTLE ORGANS / ORGANELLES
Cytoplasm
↓

CELLS
Red Blood Cell
↓

TISSUES
Blood
↓

ORGANS
The Heart
↓

ORGAN SYSTEMS
The Circulatory System
↓

ORGANISMS
The Human Being

Cytoplasm

All your cell's organelles are found floating within this gooey fluid that makes up the inside content of all cells. Think of the organelles in cytoplasm as little pieces of pineapple, mandarin orange segments, and berries floating in lemon jello. Jello just before it hardens. The bowl serves as half of a plasma membrane, if you imagine cutting the cell in half. In the cell, nothing is absolutely fixed in position; all the organelles are moving around, if very slowly. The cytoplasm is where proteins are assembled, where the initial breakdown of sugar you eat (glycolysis) takes place, and where the pH (acidity) is critical to the making of many different chemical products. The cytoplasm also plays host to a number of Antioxidants (See Antioxidants In The Cell drawing in Chapter 15).

"The Brain" - The Nucleus

Often referred to as the "Brain" of the cell, the nucleus orchestrates activities such as protein synthesis, enzyme production, and the division of the cell when the time for reproduction is at hand.

The nucleus contains a detailed description of you as well. Each nucleus in each cell in your body has the pattern for making another you. That's why the recent sheep cloning is not as unusual an event as we might suspect. We could create another you; it's just that the conditions you had when growing up would be different for this "new-you" baby. Yes, that's what you'd be making. A baby. I'm not sure what all the fuss is about cloning; we cannot yet make adult copies of people, only babies. And you can never reproduce the conditions that the cloned adults were raised in, despite the message in the films, "Multiplicity" and "The Boys From Brazil". So there will never be exact clones of anyone; assuming you believe, as I do, that nurture has a lot of control over nature.

The Plant Cell

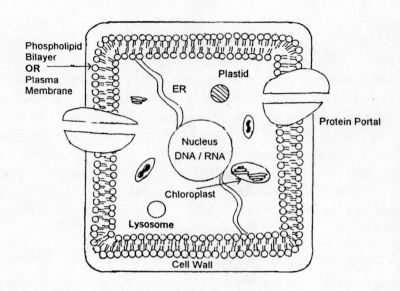

The Plant Cell

The plant cell contains all that we need to live.

Proteins, Fats, Carbohydrates, Vitamins and Minerals are found in each plant cell. Specific components of a healthy diet can be found as well.

Antioxidants like beta-carotene (in leaves, stems, fruit) are found in the plastids and chloroplasts as well as floating in the cytoplasm.

Soluble and Insoluble Fiber is found in the cell wall, different compositions in different specific cells (e.g. oats vs. wheat)

Essential Fatty Acids like Omega-6 and Omega-3 are found in the plasma membrane on the outside of the cell as well as in single membraned organelles inside the cell.

The Animal Cell

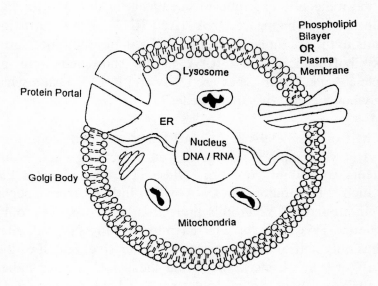

Phospholipid Bilayer OR Plasma Membrane

Lysosome

Protein Portal

ER

Nucleus DNA / RNA

Golgi Body

Mitochondria

The Animal Cell

The Cytoplasm / Mitochondria / Energy From Sugar
The organelle labeled "Mitochondria" is the place where most cell energy is produced. Sugar that is made from breaking down your food passes through the Protein Portal into the cytoplasm of the cell. Pyruvate, a compound created when the sugar you eat is further broken down, passes from the cytoplasm into the Mitochondria. It is then changed into electrons which make your energy or (ATP).

The Plasma Membrane / Fats
The fat content of your plasma membrane indirectly reflects your dietary fat. Too much saturated fat in the membrane and it becomes too stiff, cell-to-cell communication is broken down and bad things can happen. Too much polyunsaturated fat and the membrane is loose and lets anything inside; also very bad.

Transport Proteins / Protein Portals
Protein portals allow the passage of nutrients of specific size and shape into the cell. Different cells have slightly different types of these doorways for nutrients. Enzymes then attack the nutrients which are let in to the cell.

What is the molecule, or group of chemicals in the nucleus that allows all of this to happen? **DNA**. And **RNA**. Both are major participants in the continuance of life. **DNA** is the shortened form of **D**eoxyribo**N**ucleic Acid. **RNA** is the shortened form of **R**ibo**N**ucleic Acid. Your genes are DNA and RNA. That's what we mean when we say, "It's in the genes".

You get half of your DNA from your father and half from your mother. But your mother also gives you something extra...your cell contents and all of your organelles. The man donates his sperm, which is little more than DNA with a little protective sugar and protein around it. When this protective layer dissolves, only DNA is left. This DNA is injected into a living egg cell that already has only half of the DNA it needs to survive, but all of the other stuff (organelles, etc.). So while the DNA of your father meets the DNA of your mother to determine what color your eyes will be or what your favorite tastes will be, all the other stuff is predetermined by your mother. She also donates some extra DNA in an organelle we will discuss next, your energy organelle, the "Powerhouse Of The Cell". In other words, our energy comes largely from our mother, genetically.

"The Powerhouse Of The Cell" - The Mitochondria
The mitochondria are found in large numbers inside each of your cells. It's a good thing; the mitochondria are responsible for most of the energy generation in your cells and your body. In most cases, the more you have, the better off you are.

The mitochondria produce energy in high-energy phosphate bonds, which can attach or detach to or from many energy-producing compounds. The major form of this energy comes from the molecule or group of chemicals known as **ATP** or Adenosine TriPhosphate. These high-energy phosphate bonds are attached to ATP; the "TriPhosphate" means that three of the phosphates are attached to Adenosine. ATP has the most high-energy phosphate groups that can be attached to any molecule; therefore, it can donate them easily.

It is also good to have lots of ATP in your cells. Most of this ATP comes from our digestion of carbohydrate or compounds made into carbohydrate after digestion. Once we have broken carbohydrates into pyruvate in the main part of the cell, pyruvate can cross into the mitochondria. (In Chapter 8, there is an explanation of how most of this ATP is made, and three diagrams illustrating Glycolysis, Electron Transport, and TCA cycles that produce this ATP.)

Mitochondria serve unusual functions using the generation of ATP and other forms of energy. The transfer of energy takes place in several cycles, leading to the last one in Aerobic Respiration (see Carbohydrates chapter), Electron Transport (ET).

How does this energy do what we need it to? Well, the energy holders, the electrons, are sent running all over the place looking for work. When they find something that requires energy, they hook up with a big producer, Oxidative Phosphorylation (OP). This producer of ATP uses the energy of these electrons to couple, or attach, high-energy phosphate bonds to Adenosine. It's the same as if you set potatoes on top of the stove and just waited. They wouldn't cook. You have to turn on the heat! The cooking heat is actually little electrons running around doing your work for you; cooking your food!

All of this running around inside your cells, making ATP, sending little electrical charges everywhere (ET - Electron Transport) and attaching high energy bonds to your food particles with OP (Oxidative Phosphorylation) is how you stay alive. This is your energy source!

ET, Electron Transport (energy movement), in your cells is coupled to Oxidative Phosphorylation (the adding of a high-energy phosphate bond to make ATP) under normal circumstances. But a hibernating bear, for example, does not need that much ATP. So when a bear goes into hibernation, the electron transport system uncouples from the making of ATP and just keeps running, generating enough heat to keep the bear alive. This partial uncoupling is also rumored to occur each spring when skunk cabbage appears in defiance of frozen ground and frigid temperatures.

"The Information Highway" - The Endoplasmic Reticulum
The Endoplasmic Reticulum (yes, it's a mouthful) is very much like your nervous system. It serves to transport vital information from the "brain" of the cell to the "body" of the cell. A combination of this information and what's going on elsewhere in the environment of the cell allows decisions about how to respond, what proteins to make, and what enzymes are needed.

"Protein Factories" - The Ribosomes
The Ribosomes are little protein factories found in the main part (cytoplasm) of your cells. They take orders that pass down "The Information Highway" from the "Brain". These orders are very specific, but also allow for mistakes every so often; mistakes that usually don't hurt the functioning of the cell.

The Ribosomes take the information (from the Nucleus) to make the specific amino acids and then combine them into long, folded proteins. This is how we make protein and enzymes for use both inside the cells and elsewhere in our bodies.

"The Suicide Bag" - The Lysosome
Lysosomes are often referred to as "Suicide Bags" because it appears that their only function is the destruction of old or

defective cells. They carry hydrogen peroxide inside themselves and explode upon some secret command; I think there must be an oxidizing/antioxidizing function as well.

This exploding cell destruction can take many forms. One of my favorite examples is in the cells that form the abcission layer (the breakable section) on an apple stem. Upon some internal signal, from either the presence of specific chemical compounds that show ripeness to them, or a signal from the nucleus, the lysosomes in the cells in this abcission layer explode and the apple falls from the tree!

Chapter 5
HOW DOES YOUR BODY WORK?

In the previous chapter, we examined the cell and its components, the organelles. Groups of cells form tissues, which in turn are the components of our organs. Organs which work together to provide a specific function (breathing, circulation or digestion) can be looked at as organ systems.

This chapter describes some of the organ systems which are most important to our study of nutrition. Later in this book, we will examine how various nutritional habits or food-borne pathogens can affect the function of these systems.

The Circulatory System

Your circulatory system is a transport system which moves nutrients, oxygen, carbon dioxide, wastes, electrolytes, hormones, and other products through your body via the bloodstream. One part of the system carries the good stuff (oxygen, nutrients) from the lungs and heart throughout the body. The other part brings wastes to the kidneys and lungs for detoxification, removal or exhalation (carbon dioxide).

The heart is a muscular pump at the center of the circulatory system. It helps propel blood through thousands of miles of blood vessels using strong valves which open and close at just the right time. It beats about 100,000 times per day.

The largest vessels that travel away from the heart with freshly oxygenated blood are the arteries. These then run into smaller, sturdy vessels called arterioles. If the blood has to be delivered to a very small area, the smallest vessels, the capillaries, get involved. They lead to the sites of transfer of enriched blood nutrients and oxygen for nutrient-poor and carbon dioxide loaded blood. The unbroken circle leads back to your heart and lungs via venules and the larger veins.

All the food and nutrients you ingest have only two choices; to stay in your body or to leave. We lose circulating nutrients via perspiration, urine, and feces. Nutrients that remain can be used immediately or stored for future use, like Vitamin C in your adrenal gland. It is important to keep your nutrient stores up so that your body will not begin to break down other tissue, such as taking Vitamin A stored in the brain, eye or liver.

The Respiratory System

Your respiratory system includes your lungs, diaphragm (the muscle that expands when you take in air), your trachea, mouth, bronchii, bronchioles, and the tiny sacs called alveoli that transfer the new air into your bloodstream via capillaries.

Your body assumes that this new air is relatively pure and full of oxygen. That's why it goes immediately into the transport system via your capillaries. This inhaled air is taken in like an old friend, without any real screening process. There is no significant detoxification of incoming air until it reaches into the cells of your body. You and your heads-up thinking are the only screening process.

Smoking. "What's the big deal? Look at George Burns; he smoked and lived to 100." The big deal is that he probably had an unusual genetic make-up that allowed his body to aggressively detoxify pollutants entering his lungs. He was very unusual. You probably don't have such aggressively detoxifying gene products. The only way to really test your genes in this capacity is to smoke a lot and see if you end up with emphysema, lung disease, lung cancer, or any of the other cancers (like bladder cancer) associated with cigarette smoking. Before you make that decision, you need to visit either a terminal cancer home or a lung-oriented rehabilitation center.

My great aunt Freda was an exerciser, very bright and one of the sweetest people you'd ever want to meet. Unfortunately, she was also a heavy smoker. It was her only vice, really. When I was in my teens, she had a debilitating stroke that left her unable to speak well, and unable to recognize any of the loved ones that were so dear to her. My grandma Alice took her in for a while but it got to be too difficult and she ended up her life in a nursing home, unable to do anything for herself. All because of cigarettes. This could be you, if you decide to smoke or keep smoking.

Smoking, Pregnancy, and Children
Many also test the effects of smoking on their unborn children, some of whom will die, end up with low birth weight, be intellectually slower than their classmates, have serious kidney problems, etc.

I once knew a heavy smoker who loved her children dearly, but her cigarettes more. Her ignorant doctor advised her to keep smoking during pregnancy since she said it would make her tense to stop. Her baby daughter was born with serious kidney problems from trying to detoxify all of the garbage brought into her bloodstream *in utero*. The child was dead before age 4.

A second mother I knew smoked throughout her pregnancy, due to bad medical advice, and ended up having a stroke and dying right after the baby was born. Strokes are to be expected as part of the smoking sequelae. The husband was left heartbroken, with a very stressful full-time job and three kids (one newborn) to raise.

Another mother I know who is a heavy smoker has children who always end up getting bronchitis and colds. They're always sicker than their classmates. She can't imagine why. "Must be a lot of germs this year." is her standard reply. No amount of gesturing at cigarettes makes any headway with her. Too bad; she's killing her own offspring with ignorance.

Everyday we make choices for our own respiratory health, and as one health writer recently said, "Forget about worrying about cholesterol or fat; this one's a smoker..."

The Digestive System

The Mouth
Digestion begins in the mouth, with the secretion of *saliva* upon the sight or smell of food. Saliva lubricates each morsel with mucus to make passage down the digestive system easier. Saliva also contains *amylase*, an enzyme which breaks down large carbohydrate chains. Chewing creates smaller particles and the increased surface area allows enzymes of digestion to access more of your food.

The tongue assesses the amounts and types of tastes found in your food (see Chapter 24 for more information on sensory evaluation). This helps create the desire to eat or not eat. Sweet, Sour, Bitter and Salty are the major tastes found in the four different kinds of taste buds on the tongue surface. While there are general areas where certain types of tastes can be found, it is currently accepted that there are receptors for all sorts of tastes all over your tongue.

You also have the ability to perceive what sensory scientists call "Mouthfeel". This includes sensations like the carbonation of soda, the cool of mint and the hot of chili peppers.

The Teeth

The teeth, often ignored in digestive discussions, are vital to your digestive and cardiovascular health. How? As they grind and macerate your food, everything that goes into your mouth passes by your teeth or stays with them. That includes carbohydrates and sugars, pieces of fiber or gristle, and uncountable numbers of bacteria, fungi, and viruses. If you let your teeth go - by not cleaning them or by eating too many sweets - you risk periodontal disease and its potential to give you a heart attack!

The Esophagus / The Stomach

The esophagus is the tube down which your food travels to your stomach. Food is transported with a peristaltic (pumping) motion. One of the demonstrations my professors used was to show how peristalsis works in defiance of gravity. He would peel a banana, have the class gather around, hand it to one of the students, stand on his hands, and tell the student to feed him. A simple lesson, it nevertheless reminds us of the great amount of energy our bodies use in defiance of the forces around us.

Your esophagus usually goes unnoticed until it is the site of problems. One of those problems is esophageal reflux. Esophageal reflux is a disorder in which stomach acid creeps back up your esophagus and gives you distress. Acidy taste in your mouth and general upper gastrointestinal (GI) discomfort are the result.

While not terribly serious, unless acid burns your esophagus, reflux causes lots of discomfort. Two easy methods to help alleviate it are sleeping on your right side and eating less.

Your esophagus has an opening called the glottis which is covered by a flap of tissue known as the epiglottis. The epiglottis is all that stands between you and choking sometimes. It covers the trachea (breathing tube) during the swallowing of food, to prevent anything from entering your breathing system. When we say, "It went down the wrong way", we're saying that our epiglottis was not working properly. This can happen if we're talking and eating very fast. It also can happen to older individuals with more frequency because the nerves that activate the epiglottal covering of the trachea don't function as well as they once did.

The stomach begins to digest protein using acidic juices like hydrochloric acid and hormones or enzymes like gastrin and pepsin. Gastrin stimulates the flow of enzymes; the pH of stomach acid is critical to the activation of pepsin which works directly on large proteins. The stomach has an average capacity of about 1 liter. Food usually stays in the stomach for about 2 to 3 hours. Fatty meals or solid food take longer than liquids or low-fat meals to digest. The stomach only absorbs alcohol, water and a little fat. Most of the major nutrients are absorbed in the small intestine.

The Small Intestine
The small intestine is up to 10 feet long and food can remain for four to ten hours. It is referred to as the "small" intestine because of its diameter. Most digestion occurs here. The pancreas supplies trypsin (for protein digestion), amylase (for starch digestion), lipases (for fat digestion) and bicarbonate (for acid neutralization) to the duodenal area of the small intestine.

The Digestion Process

When We Eat

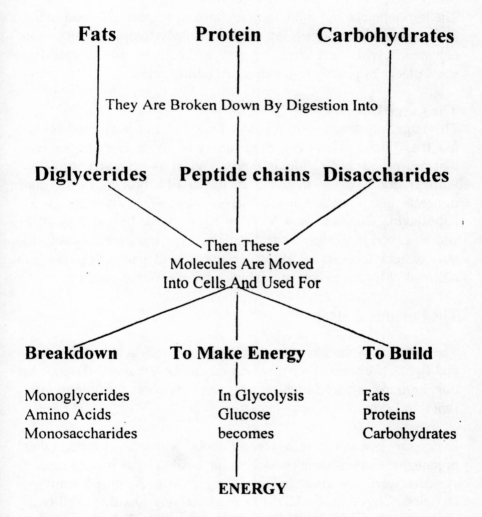

Fats   Protein   Carbohydrates

They Are Broken Down By Digestion Into

Diglycerides   Peptide chains   Disaccharides

Then These
Molecules Are Moved
Into Cells And Used For

Breakdown	To Make Energy	To Build
Monoglycerides	In Glycolysis	Fats
Amino Acids	Glucose	Proteins
Monosaccharides	becomes	Carbohydrates

ENERGY

We use this energy to grow, develop, learn, and exercise and exist.

The liver, courtesy of gallbladder storage, supplies up to 1 liter of bile (for fat absorption) per day to the duodenum as well. Bile envelopes fat droplets in a fluid for absorption.

The hormone cholecystokinin is secreted in response to food in the lower stomach or upper intestine. Cholecystokinin induces the enzymes trypsin and chymotrypsin to begin to digest medium-sized pieces of protein into individual amino acids.

The Large Intestine
The large intestine is about 6 feet long and can hold food for as much as 3 days! There is a large colony of mixed types of bacteria that are permanent residents there. Water is removed from the leftover food, plant material is bacterially broken down and minerals are absorbed in the large intestine. Vitamins B-12, Riboflavin, Thiamine, and Vitamin K are made by bacteria there and absorbed in the large intestine. The large intestine functions to also extract the last bit of water it can and package waste for removal. More than half of the bulk of feces is dead bacteria.

The Immune System

The immune system is responsible for our body's ability to resist and fight off disease. What we eat can make a major difference in our immune system's ability to perform this absolutely vital function.

Every day we come into contact with viruses, bacteria, other organisms, and pollutants which would easily kill us if our immune systems were not functioning. People with Acquired Immune Deficiency Syndrome (AIDS) have effectively lost their ability to resist diseases. They don't actually die of AIDS; they die of diseases or infections which their shattered immune systems are helpless to defend against.

There are two basic types of immunity: **Innate and Adaptive.**
We'll discuss each in detail below.

Immune System Terminology

Immunogen - (or Antigen)	A "bad" material that you eat, breathe in, or come in contact with, that makes your immune system go into "alert" status.
Immunogenic - (or Antigenic)	Causing an immune system response.
Antibody -	A flexible molecule attached to a B cell which grabs invading cells for destruction.
Macrophage -	A cell designed to eat any invaders.
Lysis -	Destruction of a cell by breaking/exploding,
B Cell -	A white blood cell that carries antibody and adheres (sticks) to "bad" agents.
T Cell -	A white blood cell which sends messages to the B cells.

Innate Immunity

The Innate immune system is the one we are born with and which protects us from non-specific invaders. These invaders are usually foreign cells, non-indigenous bacteria and some viruses, fungi and protozoans. Specific parts of this system protect against specific types of invasion. There are four major aspects to this protection.

I. Barriers

These barriers include both mechanical and physical blocks to infection. A mechanical example of these barriers is *your skin*. *Your acidic digestive juices*, and *your body temperature* are physical/chemical barriers.

Your skin is the largest organ in your body and *intact skin* is the most marvelous protective mantle that could have ever been designed. Many microbes are stopped by intact skin.

Most bacteria cannot resist the low pH of your stomach acid. It is destructive to most invaders. Once there is an invasion, we get fevers as a response. These fevers signal immune response and help us to fight invaders.

II. Residents

Commensal bacteria, found on virtually every surface of your body, serve to physically and chemically block non-indigenous microbes from colonizing. The term "commensal" refers to the type of lifestyle these bacteria live. It means that their lifestyle is such that they benefit and you are not harmed by their taking up residence. While there are symbiotic (both you AND the bacteria benefit) immune aspects to this living arrangement, it is referred to as commensal because you get an indirect benefit.

Your body is basically an apartment complex for microorganisms. Usually the tenants give you no trouble and when some microbe comes along that you think will be a bad or destructive tenant, the apartments are all filled. The times for concern are when a tenant moves out or when a tenant turns bad.

A microbial tenant can move out on you if he's unsatisfied with the conditions, like when you're taking penicillin. Penicillin and other antibiotics are like a neighbor playing loud music in the apartment complex that is your body. Lots of bacteria leave, including "good" bacteria. If these bacteria are not replaced with other "good" bacteria, problems can result. This is one reason that eating yogurt is suggested after a course of antibiotics. The lactobacilli and other bacteria in the yogurt culture help recolonize your intestine.

Your microbial tenants are changing all the time, adjusting to the environment, making changes in their surroundings. And as we age, they are less likely to perform their tasks like helping produce or digest the B vitamins. But the worst change is when one of your microbes turns "Bad". It can mutate into a virulent strain and harm you or other people who are exposed to your microflora. It can mutate with the help of healthy viruses or other dying bacteria who donate their DNA or RNA to this renegade bacterium.

III. Protective Cells
The Myeloid Lineage Cells - *Macrophages or Monocytes*
Certain cells are moving around your body all the time, looking for invaders. These are protective cells. They include *Macrophages (also called Monocytes)* which are, as the name suggests, "large eaters". These guys stick to and engulf and devour anything suspected of being a foreigner or of unusual microbial origin. They do this three ways.

Innate Immune System

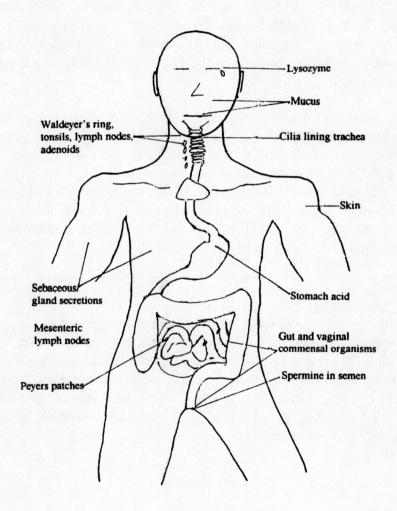

Macrophage Destruction of Invaders

Engulfment - Macrophages can enclose and devour microbes by spraying their digestive juices on them. Also called Endocytosis, this is analogous to eating.

Exocytosis - Macrophages can spray the microbial invaders with a cytotoxic compound and the invaders are digested to death without actually being engulfed by the macrophage.

Antigen Presenting Cells (APC) - Macrophages can serve as presenters of foreign or "Bad" cells to other immune cells. This occurs if the invaders cannot be handled by the macrophage alone.

Cell Receptors That Help Macrophages Do Their Job:

• **Self-Antigens** are little pieces of protein attached to the outside surface of your cells, or chemical compounds sticking out of the cells' membranes that identify them as part of your system so they will not be destroyed. This flagging of the home team is absolutely necessary since the cells of the Innate Immune System are so indiscriminate. Autoimmune disease can be a result of this system failing. While macrophages can't be everywhere to *phagocytize* or eat all the bad guys, they have help. Certain other cells serve as lookouts to send messages to and inform the Macrophages when there's trouble. And they are gourmands, as opposed to gourmets. They'll eat anything.

• **Fc receptors** are found on each antibody molecule. They grab invaders and bring them to cells that will destroy them.

• **Complement receptors** assist with the *"Opsonization"* function which happens right before engulfment. This *"Opsonization"* is a coating of the invader so that the

Macrophage will eat it.   It's like sugar coating on cereal;
sometimes they're in the mood for it, sometimes not.

The Lymphoid Lineage Cells - *Natural Killer Cells*
One of the most interesting cells currently under scrutiny for
potential immune enhancement is the *Natural Killer Cell*. *Natural
Killer Cells* are granular lymphocytes with no T or B cell markers.
(B and T cells are discussed in the next section.) Without these
markers, they do not regularly elicit help from the B or T cells, but
prefer to do the killing themselves. They are bigger than B and T
cells and are found in or near most tumor cells. The *Natural Killer
Cells* are activated by *Interferon* and other liquid substances from
the Innate Immune System.

Interferon and other substances are secreted by virally infected
cells as a cry for help. The secreted Interferons help induce a state
of viral resistance in adjacent, unaffected tissue. This is the first
line of defense against viral invaders.   These cells create
spontaneous lysis of invaders AND Cancer cells! They lyse (or
explode) tumor cells! It would be exciting if we could engineer
them to be specific and work where we most needed them.

Granulocytes **and other** *Neutrophils* -   *Granulocytes* and other
Neutrophils release endogenous *pyrogens*, or fever starters. As we
said before, fevers are very important to the destruction of
microorganisms.

Eosinophils - *Eosinophils* are responsible for helping to detoxify
allergens which penetrate the system.

Basophils - *Basophils* are also called *Mast cells*. They are
involved in anaphylactic shock responses.

IV. Soluble Factors

The Soluble Factors include Tumor Necrosis factor, Interferons, Interleukins and Lytic Enzymes. An example of a Lytic Enzyme is Lysozyme, found in tears. The evolutionary reason that we have such an enzyme in our tears has always interested me. It seems to make sense that when we get hurt and tears flow that it would be good to have an antimicrobial solution at hand. Tears suffice as such a solution.

Adaptive Immunity

Adaptive or Acquired Specific Immunity is our second line of defense after Innate Immunity. It also involves cells of the lymphoid lineage, but these cells have something special about them. They carry **Antibodies**, proteinaceous molecules which direct other cells in the attack of foreign invaders.

Let's start the story again. When a pathogen enters the human system it encounters several stages of immune response. First, the innate barriers provide physical blockage. Then the resident or commensal bacteria compete with the pathogen for nutrients and living space. Thirdly, the Natural Killer cells, Macrophages, and other Innate cells devour those microbes that they are capable of devouring. Soluble factors help zap more microbes. Those that pass through this major assault face the Adaptive Immune system.

The Adaptive Cells

An antigen arrives, passes through the Innate immune system. We couldn't fight it off with our normal defenses. Now it must face the B cells, T cells and Null cells of the Adaptive Lymphoid lineage. B and T cells are morphologically indistinguishable (they look identical under the microscope). Null cells have intracytoplasmic granules. T cells differentiate, or acquire many of their characteristics, in the Thymus gland, hence the name. B cells differentiate, or acquire many of their characteristics, in the fetal liver, spleen, or adult bone marrow.

B Cells
B cells, plasma cells, or B lymphocytes as they are varyingly called, create and secrete Antibody. Antibodies are molecules made mostly of protein, that are created in response to an Antigen or foreign invader. They are designed to chemically match the invader.

The Clonal Selection Theory is the antibody formation theory most accepted today. We feel that there is preformed antibody ready to meet invaders. The invader is tricked into selecting the antibody most closely matching it. Adjustments are made and thousands of copies of antibody are generated against the invader. These antibodies are transported through the body attached to B cells.

5 Types of Human Antibodies

IgG - The most predominant antibody in the body. It gets into all tissues. It also crosses the placenta to confer immunity to the child. Found in breast milk. Along with "Protein A", it allows isolation of Staphylococcus protein.

IgM - This is the first to arrive at the scene of infection or trauma. It has avidity (binding strength) due to its pentameric (five-sided) structure.

IgA - Found in milk, saliva, tears, perspiration, mucus secretions and in the intestinal epithelium, it protects body openings from serious infection.

IgD - The primary B-cell antigen receptor. In other words, IgD is the main antibody that picks up an invader from the B-cell.

IgE - This antibody is responsible for allergic type I anaphylactic response. Looking at what antigens cause this antibody to rise can tell us exactly what we're allergic to.

The Immune System [A Play About Life]

Prologue
Agents of destruction and immunogens enter the well-watched system daily. Vigilance is of ultimate importance. An amazing transformation takes place as the first character enters...

Act I
The Innate System Is At The Ready
A Pathogen or Allergen Enters. This invader is ready to attack a vulnerable site if given the chance. Some invaders are cloaked in mushy carbohydrate compounds for protection.

Scene I
Stomach acids, lysozyme in saliva and tears, and the protective mantle of intact skin repel the first advances of pathogens. Thousands of microbes perish. Allergens and small invaders sneak through the front lines...

Scene II
Pathogens which were inhaled are facing difficulties in an antimicrobial mucus lining the lungs and bronchii. They are also fighting to compete with the indigenous residents who have special weapons and tactics to kill invaders. It is a victory overall.

Scene III
A few pathogens have escaped; the alarm is sounded, but the macrophages and friends are lower in numbers and battle-weary. A small number of invaders escape detection and must be handled with special forces.

Act II
The Adaptive System Kicks In
The escapees have taken hold in several tissues. It is time for the big guns, the special forces. The T cells, B cells, null cells and soluble complexes. Antibody-carrying cells appropriate to the specific task are suited up and sent out. They grab, carry and neutralize most of the invaders with the help of other cells, interferon and interferon-like soluble factors. The MAC complex takes care of the rest. A complete victory!

Epilogue

Our story has a happy ending because the troops were prepared in advance, healthy and ready to fight. It could have gone the other way. Make sure your special forces are training everyday by eating enough of the right foods.

B cells have two functions; antibody formation and memory of past invaders. What good would an Adaptive immune system be without memory? If you ever encounter this invader again, it is necessary to have defense cells at the ready. The memory or Anamnestic response is critical to preventing future disease.

T Cells
T cells or T Lymphocytes are varied in their functions and work in cooperation with B cells and the Innate system. Among the various types of T cells we have T cytotoxic, T helper, and T suppressor cells. All T cells recognize the MHC or self antigens so that they do not harm your own cells, they only harm invaders. In the case of AIDS, one type of T cell (CD4) allows the virus to invade it so the virus can disguise itself as "self", and subsequently is not destroyed. So the virus has a home. In autoimmune diseases, the "self" antigen flags cells as ones your T cells and macrophages should attack.

Immunogenicity

When we speak of "invaders", we are not always talking about microbes or bacteria. Invaders can be any foreign substance which triggers an immune response. Such a substance is called an Antigen. How do we know what substances will trigger an immune response?

These individuals respond poorly when immune challenged:
Poorly nourished
Very Young
Very Old
Diseased
Stressed
Male

Factors Which Contribute To Immunogenicity

Size of Immunogen
The most potent immunogens are over 100,000 molecular weight (a specific measure for molecules). Molecules less than 1000 molecular weight will get no response. Molecules of 10,000 get a response. This means that very large molecules can create immune responses.

Chemical Complexity
Molecules like synthetic homopolymers (man-made long chains that are just a repeat of the same small molecule over and over again) will engender no response. Vegetable oil will not cause an immune response; but a complex plant polymer like the oil from poison ivy will.

Foreignness
The more foreign an antigen is, the more immunogenetic it is. In other words, an antigen from our relatives is less foreign, for example, than one from a tropical bird or exotic plant. This concept plays itself out every day in the many data banks of potential bone marrow or organ donors. It is easier, often, to find a matching relative than to search through thousands of possible donors to find an exact match. But it does happen.

Sometimes we can have an autoimmune situation where our body launches an immune response to our own cells or antibodies. Rheumatoid arthritis and lupus are two examples of autoimmune diseases. This creates havoc in the body; when the defense system literally turns on itself. In this case, you can be killed by "friendly fire".

Dose

Microgram (μg) amounts of immunogen are enough to initiate immune system response. Too much of an immunogen and we have immune paralysis. A good microbial example of this is when you expose someone to large amounts of Pneumococcus (pneumonia bacteria). There is often no response because the system is overwhelmed. If we have too little immunogen or antigen, small amounts of T-suppressor cells appear.

Adjuvant

An adjuvant, or molecule that carries the immunogen, can enhance the immune response non-specifically. It can keep the antigen from being catabolized (consumed), stimulate lymphocyte proliferation, or activate the Innate system macrophages.

Route Of Administration

This is important when considering vaccinations or contact with infectious microbes. There are three routes which create specific responses. Intramuscular (inside the muscle) administration induces a fast response. Inhalation or ingestion (breathing or eating the immunogen) favors an IgA response. Intradermal administration (in the skin) favors a T-cell response.

Health Factors

We all know that emotional factors play a role in the causes and perpetuation of disease. Psychoneuroendocrine factors affect immune status; stress depresses immune response. Aging causes T-cells to become defective. Dropping caloric intake appears to initially enhance immune response; more data needs to be looked at though. Rapidly rising caloric intake is not good for immune response.

Immune System Nutrients

A number of vitamins, minerals and other compounds have been identified as important to a healthy immune system. These nutrients are shown in the following table, along with the foods in which they can be found.

Nutrients For Your Immune System

Immune Nutrients	Sources	Function
Vitamin B-6	Nuts, Potatoes	WBC* Production
Folate	Fruit, Peas	WBC Activity
Vitamin C	Citrus, Pepper	Immune response
Vitamin E	Oils, Grains	Infectious disease
Beta-carotene	Carrots, Broccoli	Stimulates NK** cells
Glutathione	Watermelon	Immune response
Alliin/Allicin	Garlic	Antimicrobial
Zinc	Fish, eggs, meat	Wound healing, Colds
Selenium	Brazil nuts, garlic	Fights toxic bacteria
Nutraceuticals	Vegetables, Fruit	Antioxidation, Cancer

*   White blood cell
**   Natural Killer cells

Organ Systems
To Wage War

1) **Get enough cardiovascular exercise.** If you do not exercise, begin a program under the supervision of a qualified professional.

2) **Eat heart-healthy nutrients** including complex carbohydrates, folic acid (fruits and vegetables), omega-3 oils (walnuts, flax seed), and soluble fiber (oats, grapefruit).

3) **Add antioxidants** (Vitamin C, Vitamin E, beta-carotene, and polyphenolics) to your diet. Carrots, tea and apples are good sources.

4) **If you smoke, stop today.** If you don't smoke, don't start.

5) **Avoid breathing heavy perfumes** and other scents which carry volatile organic compounds into your body.

6) **Drink plenty of water.** Saliva regularly flushes out organisms. Saliva also contains Lysozyme and Secretory antibodies against common microflora and ones you've been exposed to before. The slower the saliva moves, the more microbes live happily in it. This flow is impaired by low fluid intake, anaesthesia, and age.

7) **Eat plenty of protein.** Protein strengthens your cells, helps create muscle tissue (building muscle is good for your health), and is the stuff antibodies are made of. See Chapter 7 for exact amounts.

8) **Eat some acidic foods.** Foods like garlic and grapefruit are acidic and help destroy invading microorganisms. There are organisms which can survive your intestinal acids, bile salts, and enzyme digestive defenses. These organisms can use a little extra nudge from your system with acidic foods.

9) **Utilize the Immune Nutrient List for dietary supplementation.**

INCOMING

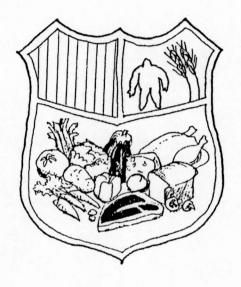

Chapter 6
FATS

Fats have been the subject of much conversation in the past few years. The amount of fat consumed is something many Americans concern themselves with. The type and the source of fat is of interest to all those who care about their bodies. Those who ignore this "fat" talk are probably eating way too much of some kind of it.

We've all heard, "Lower the fat and you'll lose weight". While this is generally good advice, it isn't quite that simple. We need some fat for our cells to grow and flourish. If you lower the fat in your diet too much, you risk serious consequences. If you consume too much, the consequences are just as dire.

Fast Fat Facts

Fats are solid at room temperature, while oils are liquid.

Fat is our chief energy storage form from excess food.

1 pound of body fat is 3500 calories.

Fat Free foods may not be Fat Free (see Tricks chapter)

Fats insulate us, absorb shocks, and are present in all our cells.

Fats help us digest important nutrients like Beta-carotene.

95% of the lipids in foods are triglycerides or phospholipids like lecithin.

Body fats can store unused drugs you have taken for years.

Beef, butter and meat fat are mostly saturated fat.

Oils are mostly unsaturated fat.

Chemical Composition of Fats

Fats are complicated groups of molecules made of the elements carbon, hydrogen and oxygen. Fats are also referred to as "**Lipids**". Some lipids are composed of three similar molecules connected by a fourth: three **Fatty Acids** are hooked together by one **Glycerol** molecule. These fatty acids can be different in several ways; length, the way they're attached to the glycerol molecule and the way in which the atoms inside the fatty acid molecule attach to one another. Three fatty acids hooked to a glycerol are called a **triglyceride**.

Fatty Acids
The fatty acids that make up the **Triglyceride** can be 2-28 carbon atoms long. (See the Fatty Acids listing in Appendix IV.) Short chain fatty acids are usually 2-6 carbons long, while long chain fatty acids are 12+ carbons in length. Medium chains are 6-10 carbons long. The glycerol molecule usually stays the same. While a Fat is a Lipid, a lipid can be any sort of fatty molecule (oil, triglyceride, phospholipid, etc.) Fats are solid while oils are liquid at room temperature.

Triglyceride
Triglyceride is another name for Fat; it merely describes, for the biologist or chemist, the situation mentioned above. **"Tri"** means three and **Glyceride** means a glycerol molecule is attached. There are also **Mono- and Di-Glycerides** (one or two Fatty Acids, respectively). Fatty acids are the simplest forms of lipids. The technical definition that food manufacturers use for "Fat" is Triglyceride. Oils are lipids that are liquid at room temperature and that are not completely saturated.

Saturation

Saturation is an aspect of fatty acids and fats that is important. Saturation refers to the type and degree of chemical bonding within the fat molecule. The three categories of fats we speak of most often are **Saturated, Monounsaturated, and Polyunsaturated**. All three have good and bad dietary aspects. None of the kinds of fat is the wrong one to eat, if done in moderation.

Saturated Fat
Saturated fat is harder to oxidize and is therefore a good defense against cancer. This means that if you have to have fat, and you don't have heart disease, you may be better off with a little butter rather than margarine. But if you have too much saturated or animal fat, breast or prostate cancer can result.

Examples of saturated fat: Butter, Beef, Avocado

Saturated fat is one fatty acid or a combination of fatty acids which have single bonds around each carbon. Carbon atoms are most stable when four other atoms surround each of them. If you look at the saturated fatty acid diagram on the next page, you can see that for each "C" (carbon atom) there is another "C" on either side and two "H"s (hydrogen atoms) on top and bottom. The end "C" has three "H"s around it. This is what we call a saturated condition.

This molecular structure causes saturated fat to be more rigid and much less susceptible to bad compounds coming to attack its integrity. Such attacks are called **Oxidation Reactions**. Oxidation of lipids is something we try to prevent both in food and in our bodies because it creates food spoilage, causes cell damage, and can precipitate cancer. When all the carbons in the fat are "happy" and fulfilled, with four bonds connecting them to each other or hydrogen atoms, there's less cause for worry about invaders.

Saturated fats are, however, very stiff...Kind of like a guy who comes to a party with his wallet in one hand and his girlfriend in the other...You can bet he's not going to mingle very successfully. It is precisely this rigidity that creates other problems for us like atherosclerosis and hardening of the arteries, and also some cancer. Too much of anything is never a good thing.

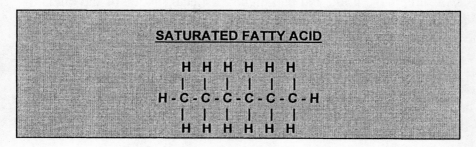

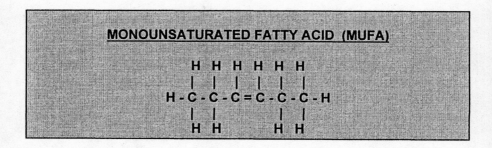

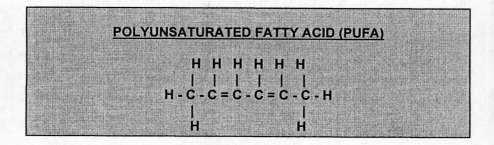

Monounsaturated Fat

Monounsaturated fat is better for your cell membranes than saturated or certain kinds of polyunsaturated fat, because it defends against cancer and disease. There is only one oxidizable site on the molecule and many of your membrane phospholipids are monounsaturated. The monounsaturated fats and fatty acids are important for cell membrane integrity.

Examples of monounsaturated fat: Olive Oil, Canola Oil

Monounsaturated fat or fatty acid has <u>all</u> the carbons happily surrounded by other carbons or hydrogens, <u>except one</u>. Somewhere along this chain there is a carbon with only three things attached to it; 2 carbons and a hydrogen (under ideal circumstances). This causes a <u>double bond</u> to form between two carbons (shown as an "=" in the diagram) and creates a bend or "kink" in the chain. It is this kink that allows the monounsaturated fatty acid chain to be a bit more fluid and not rigid enough to cause as many problems as saturated fat. An old Japanese proverb tells us to be "like the reed in the wind" and bend or be broken. Monounsaturated fats do this. A good lesson for us all. The fats in the membranes of our cells are partly monounsaturated in order to keep the membranes slightly fluid. Oxidation is a possibility but often limited to that one carbon.

Polyunsaturated Fat

Polyunsaturated fat can more easily be oxidized to set up a precancerous situation, but the necessary cancer and disease-preventing Omega 3 and 6 fatty acids are polyunsaturated! Polyunsaturates are sometimes helpful if you have heart disease and need to get off beef and butter right away, but they can set you up for cancer and possibly arterial plaques.

Examples of polyunsaturated fat:
Alpha-Linoleic Acid, Alpha-Linolenic Acid

Polyunsaturated fat is fatty acid or fat that has more than one spot along the chain where carbon molecules are not holding onto four other atoms. With carbons unhappy about the situation and willing to find new partners, it tends to be a situation easily exploited, and oxidizing compounds can come in and change the polyunsaturate for the worse. When oxidation occurs, you can have a pre-cancerous situation.

Hydrogenation

Polyunsaturates are more liquid at room temperature. One of the qualities of polyunsaturates is that they can be made more solid by just adding hydrogen atoms to the chain. This was the birth of margarine.

Great, but wait a minute. I just said that if something is added to these unhappy carbons, it becomes an oxidizing or possibly cancerous event. Well, not always, but in this case, something unusual was created called a **Trans Fatty Acid**. A trans fatty acid is a polyunsaturated fatty acid whose orientation is twisted, creating this potentially bad compound.

Heavy consumption of margarines or **Partially Hydrogenated Fat with Trans Fatty Acids** is associated with increased incidence of cancer. You will find partially hydrogenated fat or oil in just about every prepared food you eat. Look at each label. You'll be surprised.

"I don't use margarine!" you cry. It doesn't matter because you're getting partially hydrogenated fats and oils (soy, corn, etc.) in just about everything you consume. Read your bread packages, drink mixes, fast or frozen foods, cocoa, everything. You'll find this stuff everywhere. To try and avoid these takes more than switching to an organic, vegetarian diet - they're even put in packages of organic vegetables or mixes. Heads up! You must find out for yourself! Read everything!

The Three Essential Fatty Acids (PUFAs)

The Three Essential Fatty Acids
Linoleic (Omega 6) Alpha-Linolenic (Omega 3) Arachidonic

We've heard a lot about Omega-6 and Omega-3 oils lately, most of it good. These oils are also called linoleic and alpha-linolenic acids, respectively. These are two of the three essential fatty acids; fatty acids that we cannot produce ourselves. We must ingest them. They are found in cold water fish and plant sources such as flax seed oil. If they are ingested in the correct proportions, with respect to one another, there is a very protective effect. It is important to get these fatty acids in the proportion in which they occur in foods; not in pill form. The ratio of Omega-3 to Omega-6 is very important. There should be more Omega-3 than Omega-6. This proportion is usually found in linseed oil and fish.

Very High In Omega-3	Medium High In Omega-3
Anchovies	Haddock
Herring	Crab
Salmon	Flounder
Tuna	Scallops
Sardines	Cod
Whitefish	Lobster

Vegetarian sources of Omega-3

Walnuts
Soy
Linseed oil
Leafy green vegetables
Canola oil

Phospholipids

Phospholipids are basically triglyceride molecules with a phosphate group attached. There are four major phospholipids found in cell membranes.

Phospholipids

Phosphatidylcholine / PC
Phosphatidylethanolamine / PE
Phosphatidylserine / PS
Phosphatidylinositol / PI

These are used in foods as emulsifiers and texturizing agents. Another name for the lipid PC is **Lecithin**. It has wonderful properties for keeping water in products and is widely used in ice creams and gravies.

Cholesterol

Your body stores pounds of fat, but only ounces of cholesterol. This cholesterol is fairly evenly distributed among your organs. As animals, we produce our own cholesterol for body functions. We also ingest cholesterol when we eat animal products. Vegans and vegetarians who don't eat dairy products do not get any cholesterol in their diet.

Excess cholesterol in your diet can lead to a build-up on your artery walls. Sacs of it stick to different places in your vascular tree. This build-up or plaque can lead to angina (pain), arteriosclerosis, stroke, or MI (Myocardial Infarction or heart attack). Fat and cholesterol are not water soluble, so to be transported in your system they must be packaged. These packages are called **Lipoproteins**.

There are four basic types of lipoproteins. All four differ in size, buoyancy, density, and composition. HDL, or High Density Lipoprotein, is the "Good" one.

The 4 Lipoprotein Types

High Density Lipoprotein (HDL)
Low Density Lipoprotein (LDL)
Very Low Density Lipoprotein (VLDL)
Chylomicron

A lipoprotein is basically a bag of fat and cholesterol surrounded by protein and phospholipids produced in the liver. The outer membrane is a single phospholipid bilayer (see The Cell chapter) with cholesterol and protein inserted between the phospholipids. The center is usually triglycerides and cholesterol bound to fatty acids.

"What does density have to do with anything?" Plenty. If something is dense when compared to water, it will not float. Ice is less dense than water, which is why a lake freezes on top before it freezes below. Ice floats to the top of a body of water as it forms, and this floating helps any animals living in the water below to make it through the winter. Your lipoproteins have different densities, and work differently in your bloodstream. Some of them float more and help or hurt you, depending on which type you have in your blood.

Very Low Density Lipoproteins float very well. This is not good. As they float through your bloodstream, they ride high on the surface of your blood and stick to any place that will have them. Some of these places are created by injury or infection or are just susceptible to attachment. This injury can be caused by environmental insults such as cigarette smoke and diabetes or from bacterial and viral infections. Depending on the area of attachment, and subsequent attachment of other foreign bacteria and VLDLs, you could be O.K. for a while, or you could be in serious trouble. The big problems occur when the general build-up is large enough to clog arteries leading to the brain or the arteries that feed the muscle that is your heart.

When people have heart attacks, it is usually the nutrients and oxygen delivered by the blood to your heart muscle that have been cut off by clogging in your coronary vessels. It doesn't mean that all of your blood vessels are filled, just the very important ones that feed your heart. For some reason, the build-up often concentrates in those vessels.

If LDLs or VLDLs hang around and are absorbed by cells other than the liver (especially those that line blood vessels), they can be oxidized, setting up a potential plaque or precancerous situation. The cholesterol in the cells that line the blood vessels builds up and, when coupled with protein, calcium and a sheath of muscle cells becomes a growing plaque inside your blood vessels. This eventually grows big enough to occlude or block blood flow. In a person with a low-fat diet, VLDLs are broken down by lipases (fat digesting enzymes) and become LDLs. A low-fat diet also encourages LDLs to be broken down by the liver.

Low Density Lipoprotein is also very bad because it floats and is sticky. It has the most cholesterol of any of the Lipoproteins. Chylomicrons have the most triglyceride of any of the lipoproteins and are the largest and least dense. High Density Lipoprotein is the lowest in triglycerides, very low in cholesterol, and the highest in phospholipid and protein. The protein is heavy, making it the most dense package.

Typical Composition Of Lipoproteins

Chylomicron (The Largest)
Mostly Triglyceride (85%)
Small quantities of cholesterol and phospholipid
Less than 3% protein

VLDL (Small)
Lots of Triglyceride (60%)
Almost 15% each of cholesterol and phospholipid
Less than 10% protein

LDL (Small)
Mostly cholesterol (just less than 50%)
Small quantity of triglyceride (less than 15%)
20+% of both phospholipids and protein

HDL (Small)
Less than 10% triglycerides
20 - 30% phospholipid/cholesterol (more phospholipid than cholesterol)
50% protein.

The denser HDL is preferred not only because of lower triglycerides, raised phospholipids, and protein content, but because it does not float and stick to arterial walls as well as the others. There is also evidence that raised HDL can help remove some of the VLDL, LDL and chylomicrons that have adhered to arterial walls; so it behooves us to raise our HDL and lower our LDL. If the fat in your diet is low enough, your LDL will be taken back by the liver and excreted.

How much HDL should we have? Around 40 - 50 milligrams per deciliter (mg/dl) of blood. How much LDL? Less than 150 mg/dl would be OK.

A new type of lipoprotein is said to double the risk of heart attack before age 55. It is called Lp(a) or lipoprotein (a). It was found as a part of the massive, long-term Framingham study of heart disease. It was found that Lp(a) played a dominant role over levels of HDL, LDL, and general cholesterol levels. It may promote cholesterol build-up on artery walls. Low doses of aspirin, a low fat diet, and red wine may also be helpful in the case of people with high levels of Lp(a).

The biggest factor in this study of cholesterol and heart disease was smoking. According to Time magazine's Christine Gorman, "Men who light up almost don't need to worry about cholesterol of any sort. They have a much bigger problem to deal with".

Fat Facts and Fallacies

So I should eat a lot of olive oil?
No. Do not eat a lot of any kinds of fats, even "Good" ones. You'll get just as much hardening of the arteries and disease if you load your body down with olive oil fat as you might have with

mostly PUFAs or SFAs (Polyunsaturated fatty acids/Saturated fatty acids). It's just that <u>if you substitute</u> those components of a Mediterranean diet that seem to offer protection, like olive oil over butter, it will keep you heart-healthier.

We eat lots of fish and fish oil, so we'll never have to worry about stroke or heart attack, right?
Also untrue. While eating any of the fish mentioned in the Omega-3 section will offer some protection against clotting types of strokes or heart damage, another type of stroke can result! Hemhorragic stroke, where the bleeding is profuse, can result from too much fish oil. Just stick to one or two fish meals per week, or use the vegetarian sources of Omega-3 oil sparingly.

Which are the "Good" fats again?
No fat is all bad or all good, but the "Good" ones I suggest that you eat preferentially are Monounsaturated and Omega-3 Polyunsaturated fatty acids. The chart below gives the content of both these fatty acid types in each fatty food substance.

Dietary Fat Chart

Type Of Fat	SFA	O-6	O-3	MUFA
Canola Oil	6%	26%	10%	58%
Corn Oil	13%	61%	1%	25%
Olive Oil	14%	8%	1%	77%
Soybean Oil	15%	54%	7%	24%
Peanut Oil	18%	34%	0%	48%
Palm Oil	51%	10%	0%	39%
Butter	66%	2%	2%	30%
Coconut Oil	92%	2%	0%	6%

SFA=Saturated Fat / O-6=Omega 6 / O-3=Omega 3
MUFA=Monounsaturated Fat Source: USDA; Health and Welfare Canada

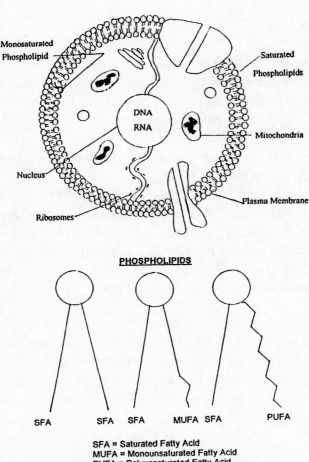

Monosaturated
Phospholipid

Saturated
Phospholipids

DNA
RNA

Mitochondria

Nucleus

Plasma Membrane

Ribosomes

PHOSPHOLIPIDS

SFA   SFA   SFA   MUFA SFA   PUFA

SFA = Saturated Fatty Acid
MUFA = Monounsaturated Fatty Acid
PUFA = Polyunsaturated Fatty Acid

Lipids In Your Cells

Phospholipids are the most common type of lipid (or fat) in your cells, but not the only type. Cholesterol and other lipids can also insinuate themselves into the membranes of your cells. An interesting aspect of phospholipids and their relation to disease and cancer is that of dietary change. New cells are being made all the time. They are being made with the types of lipids that you ingest. It has therefore been suggested that changing your type of lipid intake could not only prevent cancer, but perhaps cure it! Cancer cells rely on specific types of lipids and starving them of these lipids might result in tumor diminishment. Figuring out what lipids would do the trick is tough, however. A complete change of diet might do the trick, regardless. This is only speculation, but wouldn't it be exciting if it was proven to work!

Typical Fat Content Of Single Foods

Milk, skim 8 oz.	0.5 grams
Tofu, 4 oz.	7.0 grams
Milk, whole 8 oz.	8.0 grams
Butter, 1 Tablespoon	10 grams
Donut, glazed	12 grams
Olive oil, 1 Tablespoon	13 grams
Chicken, white-skinless 4 oz.	14 grams
Peanuts, dry roasted 4 oz.	33 grams
Beef Rib Roast, 4 oz.	36 grams

(Daily fat target is between 20 and 30 grams)

**Fats
To Wage War**

1) Eat less than 30 grams of fat per day.
2) Never eat less than 10 grams of fat per day.
3) Avoid all products with partially hydrogenated fats.
4) Avoid margarine with trans fatty acids.
5) Olive and Canola oils have the best combination of high mono-unsaturated fat and low saturated fat. Use these in place of polyunsaturated fats.
6) Make sure you get enough (but not too much!) essential fatty acids.
7) Increase your ratio of monounsaturated fat to other fats.
8) When no monounsaturated fats are available, eat saturated fat or nothing.
9) Lower your intake of saturated fat and beef fat.

Chapter 7
PROTEIN

Protein is an essential component of any diet. How much you need or desire is a function of your activity level and weight. Weight lifters often eat excessive amounts (100 - 350 grams/day) and vegetarians can get too little (10 - 20 grams/day). In general, 40 to 50 grams of protein per day is an appropriate amount. Too much and you risk serious complications like kidney failure; too little and you compromise immune and other functions.

Protein is composed of 20 different **Amino Acids** put together in an endless variety of ways. All of your enzymes, immunoglobulins, and many cellular structural components are made of protein.

The Amino Acids

Essential Amino Acids	Non-Essential Amino Acids
Histidine (His)	Alanine (Ala)
Isoleucine (Ile)	Arginine (Arg)
Leucine (Leu)	Aspartic Acid (Asp)
Lysine (Lys)	Cysteine (Cys)
Methionine (Met)	Cystine (Cyn)
Phenylalanine (Phe)	Glutamic Acid (Glu)
Threonine (Thr)	Glutamine (Gln)
Tryptophan (Trp)	Glycine (Gly)
Valine (Val)	Proline (Pro)
	Serine (Ser)
	Tyrosine (Tyr)

Of the 20 amino acids, 11 can be made by our own bodies if we get enough of the other 9. The amino acids we can manufacture are called **Non-Essential Amino Acids**. (Note: There are occasions when we need to ingest extra arginine, cysteine, and tyrosine.) The remaining nine amino acids cannot be made by our bodies and are therefore called **Essential Amino Acids**. We need to ingest these essential amino acids all the time.

All amino acids share the same basic chemical structure which looks like this:

Amino Acid Structure

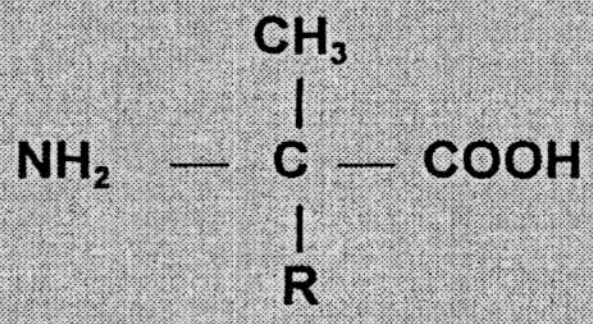

$$CH_3$$
$$|$$
$$NH_2 - C - COOH$$
$$|$$
$$R$$

COOH is called the Carboxyl group
NH₂ is called the Amine group
CH₃ is a Methyl group
R is any of 20 different attachments to the amino acid

How do We Make Protein?

Our bodies are able to create the kinds of proteins we need. First we eat the right components, proteinaceous foods with the essential amino acids. Then we break the proteins down into the amino acids or atoms that we can use.

The first step in creating a protein, once the essential components are available, is the assembly of the amino acids. This assembly gives the protein its <u>Primary Structure</u>. It is merely the number and exact order of any of the 20 amino acids. There can be all 20 amino acids in a protein or a combination of a subset of amino acids. Repeats are expected and necessary.

Primary Structure Example

Met-His-Arg-Phe-Tyr-Cys-Cys-Ala-Ala-Ser-Met-Tyr

The second step our cells perform is to fold the protein back on itself, because a simple straight line of amino acids is not very functional. This wrapping back around itself is known as <u>Secondary Structure</u>. It gives preliminary shape to the chain of amino acids (called a **Peptide Chain**).

Secondary Structure Example

Met-His-Arg-Phe-Tyr-
                              Cys
                              Cys
Tyr-Met-Ser-Ala-Ala-

The third step to a functional protein, enzyme or antibody structure is called <u>Tertiary Structure</u>. It is this Tertiary Structure that creates groups of secondary structure amino acid chains. The chains are put together into elaborate forms like Alpha and Beta-pleated sheets.

The careful assembly of these Tertiary Structures allows the final form or <u>Quaternary Structure</u> to take place. Each protein has a different and unique shape. This shape is a result of the way the

Quaternary Structure is formed. This Quaternary Structure creates **Domains** or **Active Sites** on each finished protein.

Tertiary Structure Example

Met-His-Arg-Phe-Tyr-
                    Cys
                    Cys
Tyr-Met-Ser-Ala-Ala-
Met-His-Arg-Phe-Tyr-
                    Cys
                    Cys
Tyr-Met-Ser-Ala-Ala-
Met-His-Arg-Phe-Tyr-
                    Cys
                    Cys
Tyr-Met-Ser-Ala-Ala

These **Domains** or **Active Sites** are where the action takes place. They are pockets or pouches that hold compounds that the protein works on. If the protein is also an enzyme, the active site is often referred to as the "lock", and the substance to be worked on is the "key" or substrate. These sites serve in many capacities. They are the sites where your sugars are changed; your lactose is broken down so that you are not lactose intolerant. They are the sites where the cells of your immune system recognize, grab and help devour foreign invaders. They are the sites where all you eat is converted into energy.

Functions of Body Proteins

Twenty percent of your total body weight is protein. This protein is in the form of enzymes, antibodies, hormones, hair, nails and

other components.   Dietary protein ensures the availability of
amino acids to build tissue.

Enzymes are the protein catalysts in chemical reactions throughout
your body.   They remain unchanged by the reaction, so they can
work over and over again.   In the "Lock and Key" analogy
illustrated below, the enzyme lactase is used to break lactose (milk
sugar) into two simple sugars, glucose and galactose.   If you
cannot manufacture lactase, you will be unable to metabolize
lactose (i.e., you will be lactose intolerant).   Products such as
Lactaid™ provide the enzyme within the product.

The Lock & Key Enzyme Theory

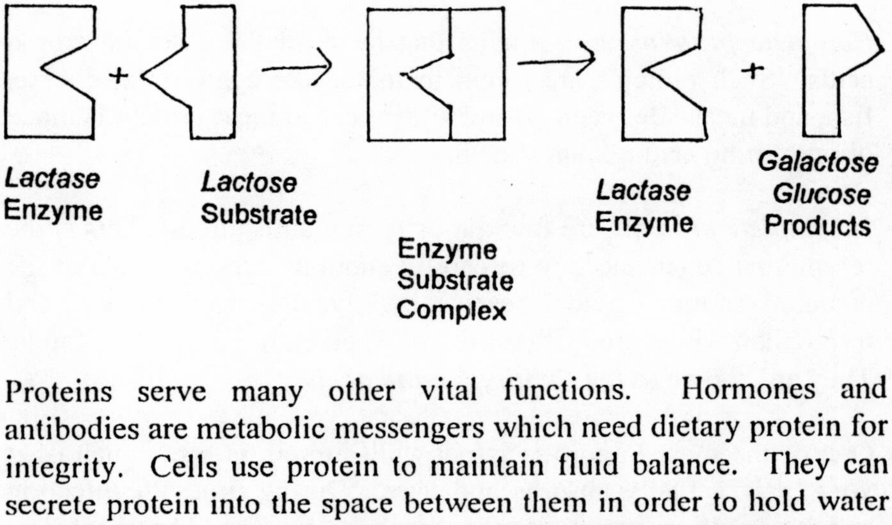

Lactase
Enzyme

Lactose
Substrate

Enzyme
Substrate
Complex

Lactase
Enzyme

Galactose
Glucose
Products

Proteins serve many other vital functions.   Hormones and
antibodies are metabolic messengers which need dietary protein for
integrity.   Cells use protein to maintain fluid balance.   They can
secrete protein into the space between them in order to hold water
there.   Proteins are used as buffers to keep the body and blood from
becoming too acidic or basic.   Proteins are also used for structure
and transport in the cell.   Some protein transport pumps can be
switched on and off as well.

Digestion of Protein

Protein digestion begins when the polypeptide chain (or amino acid chain) is broken up into smaller di- and tri-peptides and single amino acids. These are transported to the intestine where free (unattached) amino acids are absorbed. They are sent into the blood stream and taken up by cells in need. Those cells use the amino acids to make protein. If an essential amino acid is missing from your diet, there will be proteins that the cell cannot manufacture. They might be relatively unimportant proteins like lactase (without which you become lactose intolerant) or they might be proteins that are essential to fighting disease or cancer. In any case, protein production is halted. Whatever need prompted the making of that protein in the first place will not be met.

Complete proteins are proteins that have all the essential amino acids. Such proteins are found in foods like eggs, milk, cheese, fish, and meat. Between 30 and 40 percent of meat protein is made of one amino acid, glutamic acid.

Incomplete proteins are found mostly in plant sources. This is the reason that vegans need to be careful about ingesting enough of the essential amino acids, especially lysine, methionine, and tryptophan which are difficult to get when eating only plant foods. They are known as the *limiting amino acids*.

One of the most important issues with protein is how much of it your body actually absorbs and uses. During times of infection and malnutrition, you need more available protein. The *Biological Value* of a protein is measured by how much nitrogen from the amino acids is retained. The more nitrogen retained, the higher the *BV*. Egg has a *BV* of 100, or a perfect *Biological Value*. Other protein sources are measured against it. The Protein Efficiency

Ratio is also used as a standard for food labels and it suggests how much protein you might be able to use from a given food.

$$\text{Protein Efficiency Ratio (PER)} = \frac{\text{Body Weight Gain}}{\text{Grams of Protein Eaten}}$$

Protein Puzzles

How much protein do you need?
About 40 - 50 grams a day. No more. Excess protein cannot be used and the amino acids are converted to amines, then to urea after they pass through the liver, and finally to the kidney which filters them out of the blood for excretion. Excess amines and urea cannot successfully be filtered by the kidney and the organ either wears out or deposits uric acid crystals to your joints.

Henry the Eighth, for example, was plagued by wealth and diet. He had much forested land and could afford to send many bowmen out to get venison for him. As a result, he had the classic symptoms of proteinaceous excesses. Gout, obesity and kidney malfunction were the order of the day in his lascivious and non-abstemious court. Doctors at the time did not realize that some of his symptoms were the result of his eating habits and he suffered until he died.

When we eat too much protein, we also get fat. Too many amino acids are converted to glucose, then go to storage as glycogen or fat. If we eat too little protein, our blood, skin, and muscle tissue is broken down to maintain our heart, lungs and brain. With too much protein, we have a loss of zinc and calcium, raised demand for Vitamin B-6 and all of the other problems mentioned above.

I hear glutamine works for weight lifters. Does it?
It is never a good idea to take individual amino acids for the same reasons that it is never a good idea to focus on one nutrient (chromium, for example) and consume it in isolation.

Glutamine would only work if you were glutamine deficient, which most of us are not. In fact, glutamine is abundant in many whole foods; it represents 30 to 40 percent of all protein. If you really feel you need more glutamine, just eat more whole foods. Extra protein for "bulking up" works until you've saturated the system (right about at the 50 -100 gram mark) and then your body fights to excrete the excess, putting pressure on your kidneys. Eating high protein foods, especially eggs, will help you to gain muscle mass (but watch out for saturated fat!).

What about those protein powders?
You are taking a chance by loading up on the extra protein; some of these products have over 35 grams of protein in one drink! The temptation to have the suggested amount (3 times a day) is great if you want to develop muscle. You need to take all of the protein powders and carefully read their ingredients also...There are not-so-hot amounts of medium chain triglycerides that you don't want, as well as other types of "Bad" fats.

A third issue dealing with protein powders is very important. They often have no date on them, which means you should consider them <u>oxidized</u>!   Anything that is not dated could have been exposed to extra heat or time-loss of antioxidant status. (see Chapter 15 for more information on Antioxidants). The protein or the fats could be introducing cancer-causing potential into your body! This holds for any undated food you find in the supermarket or health food store!

Are you getting enough protein? Chances are, if you're eating an average American diet you're getting plenty, and possibly too much. For example, look at the protein you get in a typical breakfast:

Sample Breakfast-Protein Content
2 eggs (9 grams)
2 slices of wheat toast (6 grams)
<u>1 glass of milk (8 grams)</u>
23 grams of protein

This meal has more than half of the recommended daily requirement (of 40 grams) for protein. It would not be difficult to obtain the rest of the 40 grams in other meals. A six-ounce steak has 42 grams of protein! Any other protein you eat in excess of that 42 grams could harm your kidneys or accumulate in your joints! Or create the *Body Browning Reaction* mentioned in Chapter 16.

Typical Protein Content of Single Foods

Fruit, 1 piece	0 grams
Vegetables (4 oz.)	2 grams
Egg, 1	5 grams
Egg, 4oz substitute	5 grams
Peanut Butter (2 Tbsp)	7 grams
Tofu (4 oz)	7 grams
Dried beans (4 oz.)	7 grams
Yogurt (12 oz)	8 grams
Milk (8 oz.)	8 grams
Meat (3 oz)	21 grams

(daily protein target is between 40 and 50 grams)

Protein
To Wage War

1) Eat 40 to 50 grams of protein per day when possible.
2) Never eat huge amounts of protein for sports or weightlifting.
3) Eat foods with a protein-to-fat ratio of not less than 0.5
   (e.g. 5 grams of protein to 10 grams of fat)
4) Eat foods with a high protein-to-carbohydrate ratio.
5) Try to get real food sources of protein rather than protein shakes.
6) Vary your protein source (soy, dairy, nut butters, meat, texturized
   vegetable protein).

Chapter 8
CARBOHYDRATES

Carbohydrates are a direct result of the most important chemical reaction in the world, **Photosynthesis**. This plant physiological production of carbohydrate is so important that without this reaction, life could not exist on earth!

Photosynthesis occurs in the leaves of all green plants and algae. It is the way plants produce carbohydrate (food) for their offspring, first the flower and then the fruit from the flower. Apples, figs, string beans, oats, acorns and all other fruits, nuts and grains get their carbohydrate directly from photosynthesis. We get our carbohydrates from the fruit, nut and grain offspring of those plants.

While plants are creating carbohydrates "out of thin air", using the carbon dioxide in the atmosphere and water they've soaked up; plants are also providing the most valuable service on this planet. They give us oxygen to breathe! All other life forms depend on green plants for food and oxygen.

PHOTOSYNTHESIS
Carbon Dioxide + Water —> Carbohydrate + Oxygen

Sugars are the simplest carbohydrates. **Glucose** is the sugar/carbohydrate in the above equation and an example of the most basic unit of sugar, the **Monosaccharide**. Three common

examples of Monosaccharides are Glucose, Fructose and
Galactose. Glucose is a major source of energy for the cell.
Glucose is also known as Dextrose or Confectioner's Sugar.
Fructose is also called Levulose and Fruit sugar.

Carbohydrate Divisions

Basic Structural Carbohydrate Divisions		
Monosaccharide	**Disaccharide**	**Polysaccharide**
Glucose	Sucrose	Pectin
Fructose	Lactose	Cellulose
Galactose	Maltose	Amylopectin

Above are examples of the three types of basic carbohydrates.
Monosaccharides are single units of simple sugar. **Disaccharides**
are double units of either the same simple sugar (like glucose +
glucose) or two different sugars (glucose + fructose) as in the
example of sucrose. **Polysaccharides** are multiple units that can
be of all of the same kind of simple sugar or many different
combinations. Polysaccharides are often very branched and
"complex".

Glycogen, a polysaccharide, is the storage form of carbohydrate in
the body. When we need quick energy, we break down glycogen
into glucose and create available energy in the form of adenosine
triphosphate (ATP). Glycogen is stored primarily in our muscles
(150 - 180 grams) and in our liver (60 - 90 grams).

Fiber

Fiber consists mostly of complex polysaccharide chains, many of which are bonded in ways that human enzymes cannot break. One type of fiber is particularly good for your heart; the other is particularly good for your bowels.

Basic Solubility/Fiber Divisions	
Insoluble	**Soluble**
Cellulose	Pectin
Hemicellulose	Mucilage
Lignin	Gums

Sorting through what kinds of fiber are good can be confusing. Even the first basic designations have people stumped.

What is Soluble Fiber?
Soluble fiber is that edible material from a plant that can be dissolved easily in water. When I was just a teen, my mother would tell me things about food that it seemed only she knew. She was always ahead of the scientists of the day. When it came to fiber, though, she may have been wrong. She used to show me labels of less expensive ice creams and then Breyers. She'd say, "See all that gunk they put in the cheap ice creams? What do you need that for? We get Breyers because it doesn't have locust bean gum or carageenan in it." It now turns out that a little soluble gum or carageenan may be heart-helpful, just like oat fiber. It certainly doesn't improve the texture or the quality of the ice cream, though.

Soluble fibers are the ones that can get into your bloodstream and help with blood cholesterol and heart issues. You can find such fibers in oatmeal, dry oats, and apples.

What is Insoluble Fiber?
Insoluble fiber is that edible part of the plant that cannot be effectively dissolved in water (or even stomach acid, for that matter). So why eat it? Exactly for that reason. While it can't get into your bloodstream and help directly with cholesterol issues, it helps food move efficiently through you and increases fecal bulk. Toxins that you might ingest do not sit around long in your intestine if you eat a lot of insoluble fiber. A defense against everything from constipation to colon cancer, insoluble fiber is very important. Some examples are wheat fiber (like that found in raisin brans), and psyllium fiber (found in Metamucil™).

How We Use Carbohydrates

Respiration/Fermentation
When we ingest starches and sugars, they get broken down in several ways. Starches are initially broken by an enzyme called salivary amylase, which breaks the polysaccharides into mono- and disaccharides. More amylase and other enzymes wait further down the digestive tract and then simple sugars go to glycolysis (outlined on the next page).

If there is adequate oxygen present in the system, respiration takes place. Aerobic respiration is the term for the breakdown of carbohydrates in the presence of oxygen. Respiration is the changing and splitting of simple sugars or six-carbon monosaccharides like glucose and fructose into two useful three-carbon molecules. These two molecules in turn become pyruvate if they continue down this path.

Carbohydrate or Sugar Digestion

The digestion of sugar begins with the cycle called **Glycolysis** (Glyco= sugar; lysis= breakdown). If you ingest sucrose (table sugar) then Invertase must change it into glucose in order to enter this cycle from which we get most of our energy. If you eat mostly glucose (Confectioner's sugar) the sugar goes right into the cycle. If you eat mostly fructose or fruit sugar, it either converts to glucose (using energy) or goes into the cycle later as fructose.

Glycolysis / Sugar Breakdown

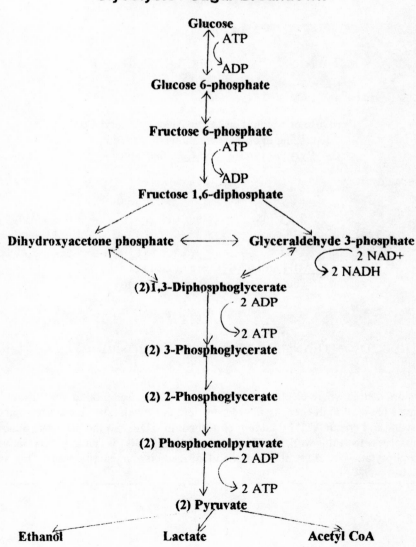

Energy From Food

When we eat food, it is converted into energy through these three steps. First food is broken down into simple sugars like fructose [See Glycolysis] and then these sugars proceed through three major steps.

Sugar
goes into

STEP 1

GLYCOLYSIS / EMBDEN-MEYERHOFF PATHWAY

and becomes
Pyruvate or **Alcohol** or **Lactic Acid**, or **Acetyl CoA**
depending upon the conditions of digestion.
Pyruvate and Acetyl CoA then enter

STEP 2

KREBS / TCA / CITRIC ACID CYCLE

NADH and FADH2 are made in Step 2.
These compounds then progress to

STEP 3A / 3B

ELECTRON TRANSPORT / OXIDATIVE PHOSPHORYLATION

This 3rd step is where electrons from the sugar are passed around very fast and create a chain of high energy. In order to store this energy, these electrons must do work and create ATP by adding phosphate to ADP. So the electrons attach themselves to this work. The work in Step 3B is called "Oxidative Phosphorylation". ATP, the compound formed, is our energy source for all activity.

In a system that has adequate oxygen, the molecules of pyruvate go into the Krebs or tricarboxylic acid cycle (TCA) where they are converted into useful energy by further breakdown.

This all takes place inside your cells. Pyruvate is small enough to get into one of the organelles in your cells, the mitochondria. In Chapter 4, we referred to the mitochondria as the "powerhouse" of the cell because it is in these organelles where most of the energy is created. Inside the mitochondria, pyruvate molecules undergo further breakdown, and in the presence of oxygen head into the last step in our Respiration equation, Oxidative Phosphorylation. It is this last step that gives us most of our energy. That energy is in the form of ATP molecules.

RESPIRATION
Carbohydrate + Oxygen —> Carbon Dioxide + Water

Why do you need to know all this? Because when you enter the health food store or even the grocery store, you are offered all the individual components of these breakdown cycles (like Pyruvate) without more explanation than, "Makes you healthy! Lose weight! Have more energy!". This information is of no use to you unless you know how these items work. And most of the over-the-counter preps don't.

There's no reason to buy pyruvate separately or to purchase any of the enzymes in these cycles. After they undergo the harsh conditions of your digestive system, they may be wasted or uselessly broken down. And who can say whether they would ever get into your cells as anything useful anyway? Whole foods are what makes your body run, not components of internal energy cycles.

Fermentation happens in the absence of oxygen and occurs inside our cells occasionally and in the cells of anaerobic (requires no oxygen) or capneic, microaerophilic (requires low oxygen) microorganisms. Fermentation is also big business. Wine, beer, bread, pickles and sausage are all products of carbohydrate fermentation. Less energy (ATP) is created. And the fermentation equation can stop at any point after pyruvate is created and a product is made from it.

These Bacteria, Fungi and Yeast Ferment And Create Foods:

Aspergillus wenti , niger
Creates citrate for food preservation
Saccharomyces cerevisiae
Beer, wine, bread
Saccharomyces rouxii
Soy sauce
Penicillium roqueforti
Cheeses, Roquefort dressing
Eremothecium ashbyi
Used to make the B-Vitamin, Riboflavin
Leuconostoc mesenteroides
Sauerkraut
Lactobacillus brevis, buchneri, plantarum
Sauerkraut and raw and fermented meat
Escherichia coli (K-12)
Microbial rennet to make cheese

Pyruvate can be changed into lactic acid (in muscle), ethanol (in wine making), acetic acid (vinegar), and several other useful products.

FERMENTATION
Carbohydrate —> Products —> Carbon Dioxide + Water

If you look at the shaded boxes above, you may have noticed the similarities between the Respiration/Fermentation equations and the Photosynthesis equation. In the ultimate design, this appears purposeful. The Fermentation/Respiration equations are just the Photosynthesis equation backwards.

Plants make the carbohydrates (Photosynthesis) and we eat them for energy (Respiration/Fermentation). In the Respiration equation, carbohydrates are consumed in the presence of oxygen (the ultimate electron acceptor), and these carbohydrates are changed into carbon dioxide and water as the energy-holding ATP molecules are made. Now our cells have energy, and as an added bonus to the green plants, we exhale the carbon dioxide that they need to make more carbohydrates for us. It's a beautiful partnership.

Common Carbohydrate Conundrums

Fructose or honey are the only sugars we should eat.
Alas, we've been led to believe that certain simple sugars are healthier than others. Generally, there is little truth to this rumor. We've also been told that honey is better than that "awful white stuff". Also not true. While there may be some extra minerals in the honey, it is mostly liquid sugar. Refined powdered sugars act similarly in body reactions with one possible exception discussed later. The "awful white stuff" or table sugar is the disaccharide, sucrose.

Fructose, glucose, and other simple sugars can all be found in fruits and vegetables. Tomato sugars are half fructose and half glucose. Apple sugars are almost all sucrose or table sugar.

What is true is that simple sugars are not as healthful for you as more complex carbohydrates. The closer you get to eating it off the stalk or vine, the better off you are. Minerals, cofactors, soluble and insoluble fiber are all part of eating a whole vegetable instead of the oil from it; or the whole fruit instead of the sugar from it.

Need another reason to eat more fruit? The Body Browning Reaction may be one. Recent connections have been made between the ingestion of fructose and the slowing of this reaction. The use of fructose as the major ingested sugar may help prevent this aging reaction.

The Maillard or Body Browning reaction, discussed in Chapter 16, creates oxidation and glycosylation, two effects associated with the aging process. This reaction requires a simple sugar, and takes place most efficiently with glucose. To prevent aging, a higher consumption of fructose (over other simple sugars) may slow down this reaction.

Carbohydrates are the healthiest nutrient.
When we lazy-watchers-of-other-people-exercising saw that the healthiest long distance runners with the most endurance "carbo-loaded" before a meet, we knew what we had to do. And the carbohydrate craze was on. "I'll bet if I eat those 2500 calories of carbohydrate all in one sitting, I'll look just like that anorexic runner..." Sure. What time's your race? Oh...

It is not the nutrient that can make you healthy, but what you do with it. Runners have very little body fat and need to load up on calories for endurance. The average weekend athlete should not try to follow a runner's diet. Nor should the average couch potato try to follow a weightlifter's diet. Diet does nothing for you, without exercise. A recent estimate claimed that some 30,000 people per year die simply from inactivity (and the ensuing medical problems). You rest, you rust.

So, while carbohydrates are necessary in your diet, carbo-loading is probably not necessary.

Carbohydrates are fattening.
So are fat and protein if you eat too much of them. Our problem, in the U.S., is not what nutrient to eat the most of, but where to cut back to match our level of activity. Yes, carbohydrates are very fattening, especially if you sit around a lot or have a sedentary job. But you can eat a bit more of them if you step up your activity permanently. Dramatically changing eating habits or exercise habits on a temporary basis is a bad idea. Gradually ramping up your exercise and lowering overall caloric intake (only if you are overweight), will keep carbohydrates from helping you store fat.

Typical Carbohydrate Content Of Single Foods

Salmon, 4 oz.	0.0 grams
Nutmeg, ground 1 tsp	1.2 grams
Popcorn, plain 4 oz.	3.0 grams
Almonds, 4 oz.	13 grams
Frozen waffle	15 grams
Raisin Bran, 4 oz.	20 grams
Applesauce, 4 oz.	25 grams
Submarine roll	72 grams

(daily carbohydrate minimum is 100 to 125 grams)

Carbohydrates
To Wage War

1) Eat Complex Carbohydrates.
The most important carbohydrates are found in whole or raw foods.
These can have soluble or insoluble components. Both are good for you
in different ways.

2) Lower refined sugar whenever possible.
Refined sugar can be found in candy, soda, cereal, baked goods, ice
cream, etc. When you use white, brown, turbinado, raw, dark brown
sugar, they are all refined sugar and received by the body as sucrose
(table sugar). Many of the brown sugars are colored with caramel
coloring which it is suggested that you avoid.

3) Get 100-125 grams per day.
It is the recommended minimum amount, though you will notice that if you
just eat the recommended minimum amounts of each of the three
nutrients (Fat, Protein, Carbohydrates) that you will have too low a caloric
intake. There is room for upward adjustment here using complex
carbohydrates.

Chapter 9
THE BATTLE OF THE BULGE

Five billion dollars each year are spent by the American public on fraudulent mail order health and diet products. Five billion! We certainly are interested in our health! It's a shame we get taken so many times by fake claims. In order to help you avoid the pitfalls of future purchases, below are some products that are either bogus or dangerous or both. These products either don't work at all or they cause you harm. Avoid them if you care about your health.

The U.S. Department of Health & Welfare has said that at least 35% of Americans are overweight. We are the most overweight country in the world. It's so bad that the District of Columbia, Maine and Illinois have or are considering a version of "sin" tax on snacks and unhealthful fatty foods. Mercifully, the FDA has decided to form the "Operation Waistline" to ferret out dangerous diets and fads that are harming the public or just not doing what it is that they purport to do. Currently, a good source of this sort of information is "Losing It" (1996) by Laura Fraser. It contains an expose of weight loss scams and programs.

Health Practices And Products That Probably Do Not Work*

Shark Cartilage
Chondroitin Sulfate
Chelation Therapy
Biomagnetic Therapy

according to any current scientific evidence

Diet And Weight Loss Products That Probably Do Not Work *

Soap for Weight Loss
Earrings for Weight Loss
Shoe Inserts for Weight Loss
Pyruvate
Vacuum Pants
Diet Tea
Staples for Weight Loss
A Juice Diet
Senna

according to any current scientific evidence

Diet And Weight Loss Products That Do Work *

Fruit
Vegetables
Low fat fish and meats
Complex carbohydrates
EXERCISE

according to current scientific evidence

Exercise And The Battle Of The Bulge

Exercise. It's a dirty word to those of us who have warmed up to the word "Dieting." We know we can lose weight if we just stop eating for a while or go on the latest diet for a couple of weeks or months. Why should we then have to exercise? It seems so unfair.

What everyone wants in this fast-paced, do-it-the-quick-way society, is an easy answer. People can follow any strict regimen for two weeks with a little self-discipline, but tell them the truth about diet and exercise and people flip out. The awful truth is that diets don't cut it and they never will. Sure, you can get into that dress for the wedding, but in a few months, you'll be bigger than you were before. Why? The rebound effect of your body conserving its resources while you tried to starve it and now overfeed it again.

We eat too much. All of us. Take the fitness quiz in Appendix I. Try the 3-day (or 6-day) diet analysis in Appendix III. What most of us find, if we're honest with ourselves, is that we are eating way too much food in comparison with our exercise. Too much energy input, not enough energy outflow. The only answer to permanent weight loss is a gradual modification of your diet to include a preponderance of fruits and vegetables, a lowering of fat, and a ramping up of your exercise regimen. A recent study of male runners who log ten miles a week found that in order to avoid getting that little pot belly we all hate, they had to increase their regimen every year. Their bodies got used to the amount of exercise they did and began to efficiently store energy as fat.

What can we do? Begin slowly to make your life better with a fun game of tennis here and there, or kicking a soccer ball with a son or daughter (or grandson/granddaughter). Play! "Play" is the operative word when it comes to exercise. We've forgotten how to play; how to have fun. Look at children. Most are not overweight. They have fun all the time running and jumping. Could there be a relationship here? Sure there is. Aside from the fact that most of their nutrients are used to grow, any extra nutrients are expended in active play.

Excuses, Excuses
A common excuse for not exercising is, "I don't have the time." Now you might remind me that, as adults, we all have to work for a living. We aren't playing all day long because we are required to

sit in front of a desk or a steering wheel or whatever...O.K. Play
when you get up in the morning. Play before dinner. Play on the
weekends. Find a sport you like and go for it. You'll live a lot
longer and be a lot happier.

Another unspoken excuse is that we'll look stupid, out of shape,
running around in short pants, trying to recapture our lost youth.
Guess again. Everyone who exercises silently applauds the
overweight woman out there trying to ride a bike again. It's the
person sitting at home eating several portions of cheesecake or
butter who is perceived (right or wrong) as not respecting
himself/herself, his/her body, or his/her family. If you sit around
and eat too much and never exercise, you care only about your
pride, not your family.

People who love these non-exercisers suffer because they will not
participate in anything. They suffer when the non-exerciser falls ill
due to his/her bad habits. And they suffer when this person dies at
an early age due to a debilitating disease or cancer they might not
have gotten had they exercised or eaten properly.

The Benefits Of Exercise
Everyone who exercises tries to get everyone else involved
because we have such an amazing secret we have to share it. You
just feel <u>SO GOOD</u> when you are exercising regularly! It is not
something you can really explain, you have to experience it. This
is why people who exercise are always trying to get those who
don't to participate.

The types of exercise that are important vary for each individual.
We all should be doing some of each of the five following types of
exercise on a regular basis:

Five Important Types of Exercise

Stretching for limberness
Aerobics for heart and mental health
Yoga/Tai Chi for relaxation
Weight-lifting for muscle strength
Interactive or Competitive Sports for team-oriented relaxation

None of the types of exercises above really supersedes another. If you do not do **Yoga or Tai Chi** moves you are missing out on relaxation that is very important for your immune system.

If you do not **Stretch**, you will get hurt, either in an incautious moment during your daily routine or during one of the other exercises. Stretching needs to be very specific; you cannot just make up stretches as you go along. Ask an expert how to stretch, go to a health club and find out or get a guide to proper stretching. (Hint: Use the Guide to TV Fitness programs in Appendix II to help you find this out at home. Basic Training with Ada Janklowitz is the best stretching show!)

If you skip **Aerobics** (which includes everything from walking briskly to competitive basketball) you will be jeopardizing your heart health. Contrary to popular belief, aerobic exercise does not have to be performed strictly in a health club surrounded by sculpted bodies and buffed patrons. Anything that gets you winded (in a good way) is considered aerobic exercise. Do your aerobic exercise by just walking up and down the stairs in your home when no one is around. There are numerous ways to exercise at home. Always consult your doctor before beginning any fitness program.

Weight-lifting. "You have to be kidding," say most people. They have no desire to look like Arnold Schwartznegger. Don't worry;

you can't look like him unless you devote 20+ years to the art of body-building. But you must lift weights! Muscle tone is crucial to your overall health and ability to burn calories. The more muscle you have, the more lean body mass you have. And lean body mass allows you to burn many more calories while just sitting!

A recent study in a nursing home revealed that it's never too late to start lifting. A research group took several of the elderly residents and started them on a weight-lifting program (even the wheelchair-bound). The results were amazing. The residents (many in their 90s and beyond) increased their strength, coordination, and posture. All three parameters improved dramatically as did their outlook on life. It is never too late to start lifting weights!

Competitive sports puts people of like minds together to have fun and get heart-healthy without thinking about it. Let's face it, sometimes exercise is boring and we are tired of doing the same old thing. That's when it's time to get a team or couple of people together to have some fun. Use the premise of a picnic or party to set up your sporting event. Any excuse is a good one.

How To Feel Healthy And Get Fit

Burn More Calories Than You Take In
It's that simple. Really. If you are of average height and weight, you burn between 1300 and 1500 calories per day just sitting around. This amount declines about 200 calories per decade after age 30. This is known as resting energy expenditure or REE.

If you eat between 2000 and 2500 calories of food per day, that's plenty. This is the recommended caloric intake for ACTIVE adults. We assume that ACTIVE adults will get up out of their chairs and burn off the remaining 700 - 1000 calories. It's not as easy as it looks, though, which is why so many of us in the U.S. are overweight.

How To Accomplish The Burning Of These Calories

By Dieting? - NO! NO! NO! Never diet! It lowers those 1300 - 1500 calories you burn at rest. And then you're in big trouble because you feel too tired to do the much-more-exercise-than-you-would-have-needed-to-do-had-you-kept-eating-normally.

By Fasting? - NO! NO! NO! Never fast! It can rob you of important nutrients like potassium, which can precipitate serious changes in your organs and organ systems.

By Eating Different Things? - YES! YES! YES! Change from butter to olive oil or nothing. Change from fatty meats to vegetarian equivalents. Change from a few vegetables to experimenting with many vegetables and fruits. Eat Indian, Japanese, Thai foods; live a little, be bold with new foods! It will allow you to vary your diet enough to make it interesting and more healthful.

By Eating More? - Absolutely, if you're eating the right foods. The more fatty, meaty food you drop from your diet, the more of the right foods you will have to consume to make up for the caloric shortfall! Never be hungry again, eat all that you want of these right foods (See Chapter 16 for a listing of the Best Foods To Eat). With heavy, meaty meals you are also really taxing your digestive system and ultimately your heart. Eat more (vegetables and fruits!) and live longer.

By Exercising More? - Oh, yes., yes, yes...Is there any other way? Nope. As the famous sneaker commercial says, "Just do it!"

How much should I exercise? There is no upper limit, except for the fanatic who is at the gym during all of his/her free time, losing friends, ignoring a spouse or children, or about to lose a job over excessive workouts. Like gambling, there are people addicted to exercise. They are relatively easy to spot if you are not one of them. Unsure? Ask those closest to you. You'll get your answer.

Exercise whenever you can. "I just want to burn off what I eat-how do I do that?" Andrew Weil suggests you walk briskly for 45 minutes per day for optimum health. He's right; it will give you great results. The list below gives a few simple ways to burn off approximately 200 calories. Figure out what your daily caloric intake is and exercise to meet it (or beat it, if you are overweight).

Ways To Burn 200 Calories

These are continual, non-stop minutes. You must be moving throughout the duration. Do not start an exercise or weight-loss program without checking with your doctor first.

Dance Vigorously for 45 minutes
Wash Your Car for 60 minutes
Swim Laps for 30 minutes
Skip Rope for 30 minutes
Play Wheelchair Basketball for 30 minutes
Bicycle 4 miles in 15 minutes
Play Volleyball for 60 minutes
Walk the stairs for 30 minutes
Walk 3 miles in 45 minutes
Garden for 1 1/2 hours

DEFENSES

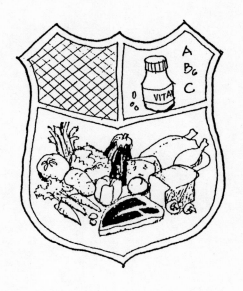

Chapter 10
VITAMINS

Why Do We Need Vitamins?

Vitamins are catalysts in biochemical reactions in the body. Without them, many functions would cease.

> **A vitamin is defined as a substance that is:**
>
> 1) Necessary for life;
> 2) Effective in small amounts in the body;
> 3) Distinct from the organism's structure; and
> 4) Not internally synthesized (Except D-3).

Vitamins are divided into two major classifications based on solubility: **fat-soluble vitamins** and **water-soluble vitamins**.

Fat-soluble vitamins are needed for all of the functions in your body that work with fats. These include steroid hormone production, prostaglandin synthesis and membrane maintenance. The main fat-soluble vitamins we will talk about here are Vitamins A, D, E, and K. These vitamins are stored for relatively long periods in fatty tissues and in the blood.

Water-soluble vitamins are important in neurological activity; some are antioxidants. These vitamins, including Vitamin C and the B vitamins, need to be replenished on a regular basis, since they are stored only temporarily. For this reason, we try to reach and maintain tissue saturation with some of these vitamins.

VITAMIN A

Vitamin A is stored mainly in three of our tissues: the liver; the blood; and the eyes. The storage levels are very important. If there isn't enough in the main storage organ, the liver, then Vitamin A is taken from the bloodstream and then from the eyes. This stealing from blood and eyes can result in problems from Nyctalopia (Night Blindness) to the much more serious keratinized lesions of the eye which result in permanent blindness. Vitamin A also functions in reproductive health, cancer prevention, and healing of infections.

Retinol and Carotenoids are the only sources of ingestible Vitamin A. **Retinol** can be found in meat, eggs, and dairy products. Many of our dairy products are fortified with Retinol or Retinyl palmitate. This insures that the vast majority of the American public will get the RDA dose at some point. However, it does not take into consideration that many people are vegetarian, that different doses are found in different kinds of milk, and that in general, lactose intolerant individuals have less absorption capability. Skim milk, for example, does not hold Vitamin A in solution as well as whole milk or 2% milk, due to its lower fat content.

The story is different for **Carotenoids**, which are found only in plants. Major carotenoids like Beta-Carotene and Lycopene are abundant in vegetable sources such as tomatoes, carrots and dark, leafy green vegetables. Beta-carotene is also found in fruits like apricots and peaches. It is generally better to get your Vitamin A from plant sources as Provitamin A or Beta-carotene. This is because there is little danger of overdosing due to the way in which it is absorbed. Provitamin A is the precursor to Vitamin A. It only needs to be split correctly in the body to release Vitamin A.

We have an enzyme called Beta-carotene 15-15' Dioxygenase which splits the Beta-carotene molecule into the equivalent of two Vitamin A molecules. (This, by the way, is one of my arguments to prove that humans were initially herbivores. Carnivores do not have this enzyme!) Since nothing is ever perfect, we usually absorb the equivalent of little more than one of those Vitamin A's.

Like all of our enzymes, there is only so much Beta-Carotene 15-15' Dioxygenase to go around. The amount we have available at any one time is determined by our current level of tissue-stored Vitamin A. Much of our beta-carotene is stored in organs such as the fovia of the eye and in the ovary. If we are in need of Vitamin A, there will be more of this carotenoid-splitting enzyme available. If we have enough stored Vitamin A, there will be less of it available.

Vitamin A comes in three separate forms:

Retinol
Retinal
Retinoic Acid

In the standard vitamin preparation, Vitamin A (as **Retinol**) is attached to acetate or palmitate to stabilize it for absorption. **Retinol** is the form that is most easily absorbed from ingestion. It is **Retinoic Acid** that is often used in acne treatments or topical wrinkle removal cream. Although some **Retinoic Acid** is absorbed through the skin, it is not stored in the liver, blood or eyes like the other forms.

Vitamin A

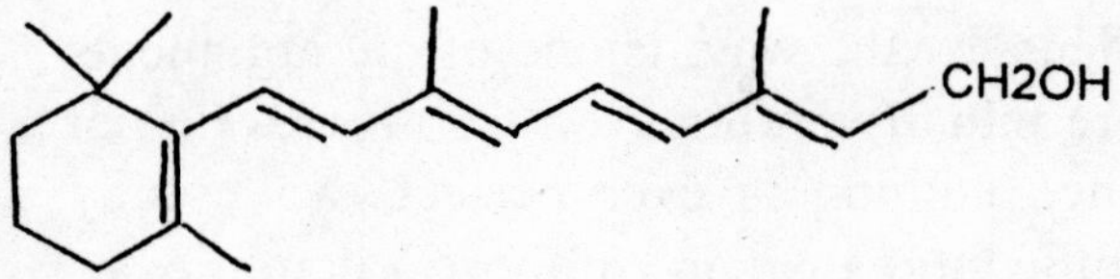

Retinol

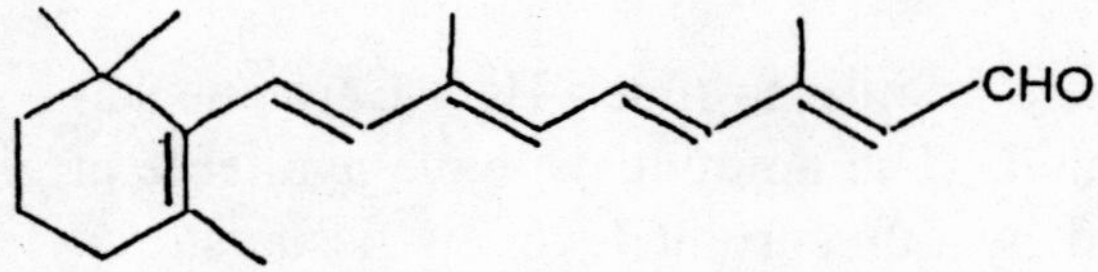

Retinal

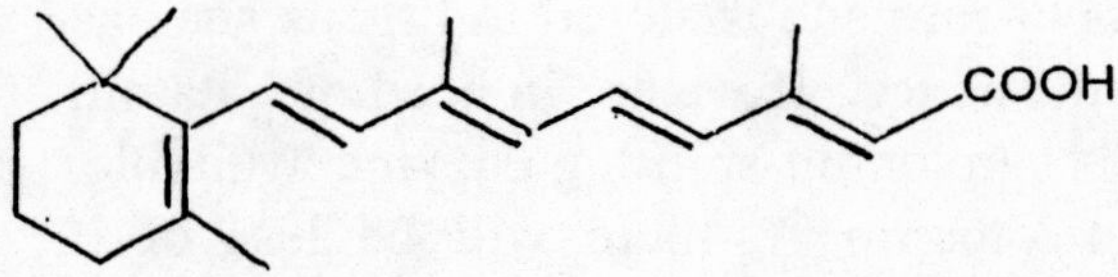

Retinoic Acid

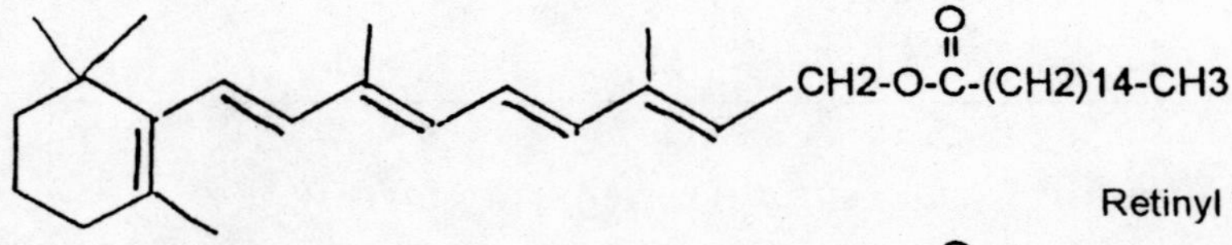

Retinyl Palmitate

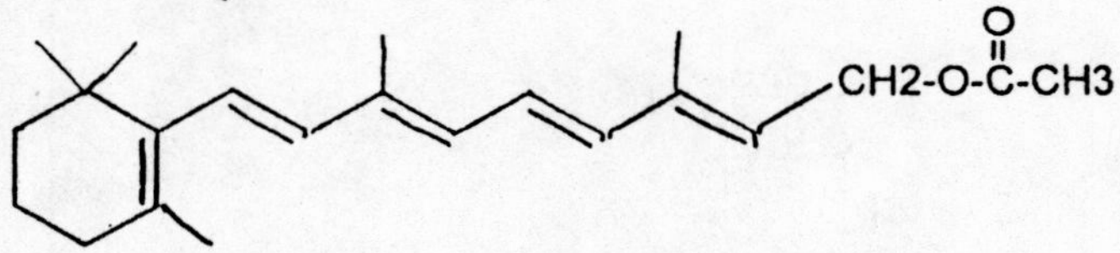

Retinyl Acetate

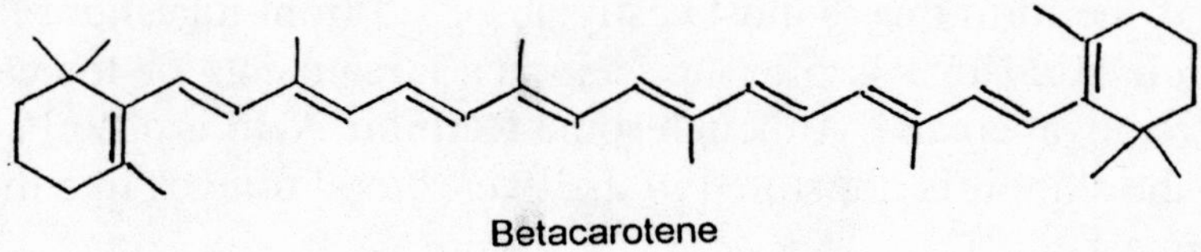

Betacarotene

Symptoms of Vitamin A Deficiency

EYE
Nyctalopia (Night Blindness)
Xerosis (Dryness of the eye)
Bitot's Spots (on eyeball surface; indicative of deficiency)
Xerophthalmia (Atrophy and dullness to eye)

SKIN
Metaplasia (precancerous change in cell structure)
Hyperkeratinization (Cornification or rough, horny skin)
Desquamation (shedding of outer rough layers)

REPRODUCTIVE SYSTEM
Irregular Estrus (female)
Sterility (male)

INFECTIONS
Urolithiasis - calculi of keratinized skin(stones in kidney)
Dry Openings allow numerous infections

Recommended Dietary Allowance
4000 International Units (IU) per day for women; 5000 IU per day for men.

Toxicity
Too much Vitamin A can result in a toxic syndrome which causes reproductive problems including birth defects.

THE B VITAMINS

The B vitamins work in concert. When there is a deficiency or oversupply of one, it can precipitate deficiency or oversupply of another. The B vitamins also work with other water soluble vitamins. Too much B-12 works against the Vitamin C concentrations in your tissues, and too much Vitamin C prevents absorption of B-12.

The B vitamins are also **Co-enzymes**, which means that without their input, certain enzymatic reactions will not take place. They allow enzymes to work; to break down sugars, to form high energy bonds, etc. This is why you will hear that you need B vitamins for energy. While they do not provide energy specifically, they are catalysts for its use. The major co-enzymes are TPP (Thiamine), FMN/FAD (Riboflavin), and Pantothenyl CoA (Pantothenate).

VITAMIN B-1 (Thiamine)

Thiamine was the first vitamin to undergo rigorous study. In the early 1900's in Java, natives who only consumed rice acquired mysterious symptoms. Their knees shook, their feet and hands became numb and they walked with an unusual gait. The Javanese referred to this disease as "Sheep walk" or Beriberi.

It was a Japanese naval captain who realized that his men who consumed no only rice on a long mission, got Beriberi. He compared these men to those who ate a variety of foods (green peas, meat, and other vegetables) and were protected from Beriberi. The good doctor then supplemented the diets of all sailors and eliminated the problem.

One of the problems with the over-processed food supply in the U.S. is that we eventually have to add back the vitamins we've removed. Such is the case with rice. Polished rice, such as we get in the U.S., has had the B vitamins removed through the polishing process; they are usually added back at a later stage of processing. This is why you should eat unprocessed, less-processed, or brown rice wherever possible.

Symptoms of Vitamin B-1 (Thiamine) Deficiency

Infantile Beriberi
Characterized by a loud piercing cry followed by an aphonic (soundless) cry. Cardiac arrest is possible. This condition is present in infants 2-6 months who are breast-fed by thiamine-deficient mothers. There is abdominal distention, and malabsorption may lead to anorexia. Infants often just stop eating and cannot be forced to resume.

Wet Beriberi
Enlarged heart, peripheral edema, or cardiac failure can result from this condition. Caloric intake is good, unlike the infantile syndrome.

Dry Beriberi
Protein/calorie malnutrition results in peripheral wasting of the lower limbs and neurological symptoms such as lack of feeling or partial paralysis.

Wernicke-Korsokoff Syndrome
Alcoholics often develop the symptoms of B vitamin deficiencies, especially Thiamine deficiency. These symptoms include the characteristic gait of Beriberi, memory failure, nervousness, and sleeplessness. Patients can appear uncooperative, confused and may go into coma as a result. One of the most interesting symptoms is an unusual nystigma (eye movement) where the eyes go back and forth like the person is watching a train go by. This problem can be solved in its early stages with intervention and administration of Thiamine, provided there are no other B vitamin deficiencies.

Without thiamine, we can't make fatty acids and our nucleic acid generating capability goes down. We need the ability to make fatty acids and have cell division so our tissues can regenerate themselves. This requires nucleic acid formation. The average thiamine-deficient person loses weight (in a very unhealthy way) and has symptoms similar to a malnourished alcoholic.

Recommended Dietary Allowance
1.5 milligrams (mg) daily

VITAMIN B-2 (Riboflavin)

Riboflavin was discovered by two scientists simultaneously, while trying to break down Glucose-6-Phosphate. Why is this of interest? Well, if you look at the drawings of the breakdown of foods and sugars (see the glycolysis diagram in Chapter 8), you will understand that you would get no energy from glucose without enzyme activity! An enzyme is required at each "arrow" in the reaction. And you can also see that the B vitamins play an important role in this energy production in that food breakdown cycle.

Riboflavin is found in the body as Flavin Adenine Dinucleotide (FAD) or Flavin Mono Nucleotide (FMN) in this form. The FAD and FMN are essential to maintaining energy in the cells of your body. They hold and transport energy produced by the breakdown of foods.

The upper portion of the small intestine absorbs riboflavin (except for any produced by the bacteria in the large intestine which is absorbed there) and it is better absorbed if taken with food. It is a saturable absorption system, meaning that the body will only take up as much as needed if given a large supply.

In certain enzyme reactions Riboflavin is critical. Riboflavin is used in fatty acid oxidation to break off two carbon units at a time. Several enzyme reactions like cytochrome reductase also need FAD/FMN.

At low intakes, ATP (see Chapter 8 on carbohydrates) and sodium (Na++) are needed to facilitate riboflavin uptake. Uremia (a kidney condition), antacids and high fiber inhibit absorption of riboflavin. Riboflavin, once in the body, is bound to albumin (a protein with weak hydrogen bonds), IgG (Immunoglobulin G - see Immune System section of Chapter 5), riboflavin binding protein, and other proteins. Pregnant mammals have lots of riboflavin binding protein. This binding to proteins helps prevent kidney loss of this valuable, water-soluble nutrient, but it does not help transport it to where it is needed.

Cells of the kidney and liver are the most efficient at uptake of riboflavin. It is stored in the liver as FAD (up to 1/3 of the body supply) and in high concentrations as free, unbound riboflavin in the retina. It can, however, be found in all body cells. Riboflavin, like Thiamine, is metabolically trapped in cells because it is phosphorylated (has a Phosphorus attached).

The most important function of riboflavin is the energy component. Without riboflavin changing into FAD, high amounts of fat, carbohydrate or protein will give you little energy. Why? Because riboflavin in the diet allows the transport of electrons through the Electron Transport Chain. It is this transport that gives our final needed dose of ATP, the energy-giving molecule.

It is important that your body convert the riboflavin you ingest into FAD and FMN. The half-life of riboflavin in the body is 16 days. We lose 0.2 mg/day in urine and feces if we have a normal intake. Riboflavin provides urine with that characteristic yellow color after we take a multiple vitamin or a mega-B supplement. Riboflavin is important in antioxidant status and DNA synthesis.

Symptoms of Vitamin B-2 (Riboflavin) Deficiency

Failure to thrive (infants)
Lack of growth
Glossitis (red, swollen tongue--flat pilli)
Loss of taste
Swollen lips
Paralysis
Estrus cycle ruined
Sebborrheic dermatitis
Collagen maturation impaired (can't heal wounds)
Skin problems aggravated by high fat diet because of defect in fatty acid breakdown

Larger amounts of Riboflavin needed in:

Hyperthyroidism
Diabetes
Alcoholism
Chronic Stress
Pregnancy
Elderly patients
Beta-thalassemia (FMN--X--FAD)
Biliary atresia
Phototherapy for jaundice in newborns
Thorazine therapy (Chlorpromazine)
Dialysis
G6PDH deficiency (less FMN, more FAD)

Recommended Dietary Allowance
1.7 milligrams (mg) daily

VITAMIN B-3 (Niacin)

There are three forms of Niacin commonly found in the body, NAD (Nicotinamide Adenine Dinucleotide), NAM (Nicotinamide), and NA (Nicotinic Acid or Niacin). We are able to synthesize Niacin from the amino acid Tryptophan in our cells. 60 milligrams of Tryptophan is equivalent to 1 milligram of Niacin. You may recognize one or more of these forms of Niacin if you know someone with dangerously high cholesterol. Niacin is used as the emergency and short-term treatment for high cholesterol (300+). Niacin inhibits the lipolysis (or breakdown) of fat in adipose tissue. This results in the lowering of VLDL, LDL, cholesterol, triglycerides, and free fatty acids created from your fat or adipose cells. It also raises your HDL. It doesn't address your fat intake, though. You need to do that yourself (see Chapter 6).

Why can't you medicate yourself with Niacin if you suspect that your cholesterol is high? You can. However, you should do so only by eating natural niacin sources like enriched grains, mushrooms, peanuts or tuna and chicken, or by enhancing the level of tryptophan in your system with milk or turkey. Do not take high-dose supplements. Many of these give you 1000+% of your daily requirement; you only need 100% every three days or so. Taking supplements can also be dangerous, and the cholesterol-lowering effect lasts only while you're taking Niacin. As soon as you stop taking it, there is a rebound to dangerous levels unless you've changed your diet and lifestyle.

Deficiency Symptoms
Most B vitamins have similar deficiency symptoms, called the "four Ds". Deficiency can be serious enough to cause death, but this is rare in developed countries. Inborn errors of metabolism (Hartnup's disease), Carcinoid syndrome (where tryptophan is

catabolized by a minor biochemical pathway), and tumors that change tryptophan to seratonin can help create deficiency symptoms.

> **The Four "D"s**
> Diarrhea
> Dermatitis
> Dementia
> Death

Besides these symptoms of Niacin (and other B vitamin) deficiencies, there is the major disease Pellagra. Pellagra is characterized by weakness, anorexia, indigestion and wasting.

Recommended Dietary Allowance
6.6 milligrams per 1000 calories, or 15 - 19 milligrams total, daily. The average daily diet has 16 - 34 milligrams of Niacin.

Toxicity
Itching and flushing of the skin are typical symptoms of high doses of Niacin. Care needs to be taken that more serious symptoms do not develop, so a physician should be apprised of your "Niacin flush" if you get one.

VITAMIN B-6 (Pyridoxine)

Vitamin B-6 is vital for nutrient processing, serving as a coenzyme in reactions involving amino acids and protein. In one such reaction, it helps to convert homocysteine (which can damage blood vessel linings) into methionine. Vitamin B-6 may also increase the synthesis of seratonin, important in many functions.

Deficiency Symptoms
Circulating protein levels are reduced.

Recommended Dietary Allowance
2 milligrams daily. This RDA corresponds to a daily protein intake of 126 grams, which is significantly more than you need.

Toxicity
Daily doses of 2 grams (2000 milligrams) can lead to nerve damage, walking difficulties, and numbness in the extremities.

VITAMIN B-12 (Cyanocobalamin) / FOLATE

Vitamin B-12 functions as an important coenzyme in the body, in fatty acid catabolism (breakdown), nervous system myelination (covering over nerves) and in the reduction of glutathione.

Folate helps to transfer carbon atoms from one compound to another. Tetrahydrafolate (THF) is the folate vehicle of transfer. If you take oral contraceptives, you may occasionally have an abnormal Pap smear or changes in the cervical epithelium; folate (and sometimes Beta-carotene) can help correct those changes that are strictly due to the oral contraceptives.

Note
Any abnormal Pap test should be looked at twice; by two different doctors. Don't try to cure yourself with vitamins or herbs. And never rely on just one opinion. A 24 year old co-worker of mine (a heavy smoker with condyloma warts) was very weak, had an abnormal smear (dysplasia) and was bleeding irregularly and heavily and she had only one doctor. I knew she probably had advanced cervical cancer. "He's the doctor; he knows what's going on..." was what she said to me when I questioned the wisdom of his scraping part of her cervix several times over weeks to test it. "You need to have it removed now! Get another

opinion!" I urged her. She said she didn't want to give up the possibility of having children because her boyfriend wanted to marry her. Instead, one month later, she gave up her life.

Deficiency Symptoms

Vitamin B-12: Deficiency is often associated with age, alcohol consumption, gastrointestinal surgery, and vegetarianism. This deficiency can be an error in propionate metabolism, microcytic hypochromic anemia, or macrocytic anemia. In another disorder related to Vitamin B-12, megaloblastic anemia, it is hard to discern between Vitamin B-12 and Folate deficiency.

Folate: Most of our folate is stored in the liver. THF carries its one carbon from the amino acid serine to other compounds that need it. One of those compounds is our nucleic acid or DNA. A deficiency shows in inefficient DNA synthesis, megaloblastic cells, and abnormal red blood cells and epithelial cells (e.g. cervical cells). Cancer drugs like methotrexate inhibit folate reactions and absorption. A major symptom in pregnant women is neural tube defect in their fetuses.

Homocysteine, an "aberrant" amino acid, has become an important diagnostic compound in the assessment of heart disease. If it is high, there is a danger of hidden heart disease. Many heart disease patients have heat-labile THF, meaning that this folate product cannot work in their cells. It is necessary to have a sufficient and steady supply of folic acid (by eating fruits and vegetables) so that too much homocysteine is not produced and other important body functions are not sacrificed. To avoid these effects, eat fresh fruit on a regular basis. Supplementation can be used sparingly and occasionally. The best, most bioavailable source of folate is lima beans, both cooked and frozen.

Recommended Dietary Allowance
B-12: 2 - 3 micrograms per day
Folate: 200 micrograms per day

Toxicity
Vitamin B-12: We hang on to our B-12 for years. It is not necessary to supplement it because we usually get it in our food. While not toxic, more than the (up to) 20 micrograms we ingest per day via food is not necessary except in the elderly who suffer deficiencies.

Folate: Epileptics who take Phenytoin (an analog of folate) can get convulsions with folate. Insomnia and general malaise can result as well, but there is very little toxicity.

VITAMIN C (Ascorbic Acid)

Most mammals cannot synthesize Vitamin C. Possible exceptions are guinea pigs and dogs, although we are now finding out that dogs need Vitamin C. And contrary to popular belief, both the B-vitamins and Vitamin C ARE stored in the body! We have been told that the "water-soluble" vitamins need to be replenished every day because they are not stored like the fat-soluble ones. It's just not true. Vitamin C is taken up by our CNS (Central Nervous System), our leukocytes (white blood cells), and our adrenal and pituitary gland (where Vitamin C is stored).

Vitamin C functions as an antioxidant in concert with Vitamin E, in collagen formation, wound healing, and blood vessel health. Vitamins C and E work with the enzyme that breaks down Beta-carotene so that it's useful in the body as Vitamin A. Animals with low Vitamin C do not make defective collagen, they just make less of it. Without Vitamin C, we lose the ability to regenerate Vitamin

E and glutathione after they help with antioxidant functions. Without Vitamin C we have low adrenalin functions and low energy. Vitamin C helps detoxify steroids, drugs, and heavy metals. It can help you recover faster from the effects of chemotherapy as well.

Vitamin C was found to be necessary after British sailors who were out to sea for months developed Scurvy (a blood vessel weakening). Easily bruised, weak, and having low resistance to infection, the sailors needed something. When they stopped in a tropical port and consumed limes and lemons, all their symptoms disappeared. Henceforth they carried limes with them on every sail and became known as "Limeys".

Symptoms of Vitamin C Deficiency

An unusual list of what initially appear to be disparate symptoms characterize Vitamin C deficiency. They are referred to as the "4 'H's".

The 4 "H"s
Hemorrhagic problems
Hyperkeratosis
Hemolytic problems
Hypochondria

Other symptoms include:
Scurvy--characterized by bleeding gums and excessive bruising
Connective tissue problems
Depression
Petechiae (little blood spots under the skin)
Arthralgia (joint effusions)
Fatigue
Anemia
Follicular hemorrhage (red ring around hair follicle)
Low resistance to infection

Recommended Dietary Allowance
While the RDA of Vitamin C is 60 milligrams per day, we really need about 75 milligrams per day to keep the storage pool constant. Smokers need a little bit more to guard against the oxidizing effects of the contaminants in cigarette smoke. There are some who advocate huge daily doses of Vitamin C (5,000 - 10,000 milligrams per day), but that is dangerous and excessive. At these levels you run the risk of blocking the absorption of other critical nutrients. I recommend never taking more than 250 milligrams at any one time.

Toxicity
Excessive Vitamin C in your urine can result in oxalate stones in your kidneys. Some organs will sequester or store excessive amounts as well. This could result in an imbalance of other nutrients.

VITAMIN D

Vitamin D functions in several different systems. Its most important function is to help maintain a constant level of calcium in your blood. Even a small deviation in blood calcium can result in death. Vitamin D facilitates absorption and transport of calcium in the intestine, if we get enough calcium in our diet. If we are not eating enough calcium, Vitamin D can assist the body with decalcifying stored calcium in our bones.

Vitamin D is stored in fish liver. We store Vitamin D in muscle tissue and blood (not as much in our liver). Tuna fish liver is one of the best sources. Remember when moms used to make their children drink cod liver oil? They consumed it for this reason (along with Vitamin A and essential oils). We don't recommend cod liver oil anymore because the concentration of vitamins is so high it could be toxic.

Our need for Vitamin D depends on a variety of factors.

Factors That Determine Need For Vitamin D
Quantity ingested
Length of insolation (exposure to sunlight)
Season
Time of Day/Location
Clothing
Skin color (amount of melanin)

We can manufacture Vitamin D in sufficient quantities if we receive enough sunlight. In the summer, we can make 6 International Units (IU) of Vitamin D-3 per square centimeter of skin per hour. In the winter, we make about one quarter of this amount. Two hours of sunlight gives 200 IU (5 micrograms) on your face alone; enough for a daily dose. The wavelength 305λ seems to be optimal for conversion.

There are two types of Vitamin D. **Ergocalciferol** (Vitamin D-2) is obtained from plant sources, while **Cholecalciferol** (Vitamin D-3) is animal-based.

Ergocalciferol (Vitamin D-2)
Ergosterol is the most abundant plant sterol. It becomes Ergocalciferol in the body. It can be found in the leaves of day-blooming *Jesamine* and *Solanum malcoxylon*, the bread and wine yeast *Saccharomyces cerevisiae*, and in *Aspergillus niger,* the fungus used in food production. Only humans appear to be able to use Vitamin D-2.

Cholecalciferol (Vitamin D-3)

7-dehydrocholesterol (pro D-3) becomes cholecalciferol (Vitamin D-3). The induction of 7-dehydrocholesterol into Vitamin D-3 requires insolation (the action of the rays of the sun). When we eat animal products, we are ingesting already-formed Vitamin D-3. When we sit in the sun, we are making our own Vitamin D-3 from 7-dehydrocholesterol. When we ingest plant ergocalciferol (Vitamin D-2), we have ready-made Vitamin D. Food scientists synthesize Vitamin D or irradiate yeast or other material with UV light to make Vitamin D-2 to fortify our dairy products, even though there is a natural level of Vitamin D in milk. Go figure.

Deficiency Symptoms

Osteomalacia, demineralized bone and decalcification to soft bones, is one of the results of lack of Vitamin D. We mentioned earlier that calcium concentration in the blood never changes. That is why it is useless to try to determine your body's calcium status by simply measuring blood levels. Without enough Vitamin D to process the calcium we eat, the body begins to cannibalize its internal calcium reserves to keep blood calcium levels up.

In extreme cases of Vitamin D deficiency, the calcium concentration in our blood falls, and our bodies fight to scavenge any remaining calcium, including that which is stored in muscle tissue. The result is Tetany, a condition in which muscles freeze and cannot relax. This condition is often fatal.

Without calcium, blood will not clot, but a person will die of tetany long before their blood loses its clotting ability.

Recommended Dietary Allowance

Between 200 and 400 IU (5 to 10 micrograms) daily.
1 IU of Vitamin D equals 0.025 micrograms.

Toxicity

Vitamin D is a hormone and a poison because of its action, but it is hard to get too much from food. It works together with the kidney, liver, and parathyroid gland for regulation. False testosterone, estradiol, and progesterone all play a role in absorption of calcium via Vitamin D induction. If you drink a lot of milk, you might want to contact the dairy and ask exactly how much Vitamin D is put in each half gallon. It turns out that different manufacturers put different amounts into their milk. This can cause toxicity or deficiency if you're not careful.

Do not take Vitamin D supplements. Quantities in the range of 1,000 to 2000 IU are very toxic. Also pay attention when dealing with baby foods, especially if you mix them. Each jar of baby food usually has 100% of the baby's daily dose.

Symptoms of toxicity can include painful calcium crystals in liver, blood vessels, kidneys and heart. Excess Vitamin D restricts organ action and creates bone outgrowths. These conditions are reversible if caught early.

VITAMIN E

Vitamin E was discovered when animals without it gave birth to offspring with muscular dystrophy, and a failure to thrive. "Tocopherol", the name given to the vitamin, means "to bring forth birth". Vitamin E may also serve us well in the fight against cancer, heart disease and Altzheimer's disease. There are suggestions of benefits in several categories, but because there is no real deficiency syndrome, it is a very under-studied vitamin.

A most interesting recent suggestion is that Vitamin E has great antioxidant power. Vitamin E helps sequester and metabolize iron in the cell, as well as improve Vitamin A absorption when the supply of Vitamin A is low. It keeps platelets from clumping and may keep LDLs from oxidizing.

Deficiency Symptoms

Without adequate Vitamin C, recycling of Vitamin E cannot occur and deficiency can result. In red blood cell membranes, which are sensitive to oxidizing compounds, breakdown (hemolysis) can result. Heart disease and cancer may be long term results as well.

Recommended Dietary Allowance

30 International Units (IU) per day is suggested, but higher doses (200 IU/day) may have significant preventative effects. 200 - 400 IU per day is suggested for post-menopausal women. 400 IU is too high to take on a regular basis and may raise your blood pressure if you're not used to it.

Toxicity

Too much Vitamin E can cause headaches, nausea, and fatigue. It can also compromise Vitamin K status, which can be dangerous if you're on blood thinners or anticoagulant compounds.

VITAMIN K

Vitamin K is so named because it affects "koagulation" (a Danish term) of blood. It serves to activate blood clotting factors. The best Vitamin K sources are yellow and green leafy vegetables, fish oil and meat.

The Three Types of Vitamin K

Phylloquinone (K-1) - Found in plants
Menaquinone (K-2) - Found in microbes
Menadione (K-3) - Found in animals

Deficiency Symptoms
People who are on long-term antibiotic usage or who have severe
fat malabsorption can have a deficiency of Vitamin K. Blood
clotting problems are one result of the diminished capacity of
intestinal bacteria to manufacture Vitamin K. In other words,
hemorrhages are possible if you don't eat your green veggies. This
is one more reason that it is very important for children to eat their
vegetables.

Recommended Dietary Allowance
60-80 micrograms per day.
The average U.S. diet can have 300-600 micrograms per day, so
Vitamin K deficiency is uncommon.

Toxicity
Because it is readily excreted and found mostly in vegetables, there
is little chance for toxicity. Toxicity symptoms can include excess
prothrombin (a blood-clotting protein) because Vitamin K helps
synthesize it. This might create excess clotting, but is unlikely.

SUMMARY

The table below summarizes the important vitamins, their sources,
and target values for consumption. The listed target values are
typical for normal, healthy adults. Additions or restrictions may be
appropriate, but should be implemented only upon the advice of a
qualified professional.

Most people feel the temptation, when they learn of a new vitamin
or other health-promoting compound, to run down to the
supermarket or health food store and buy the miracle drug in pill
form. Most Americans take some sort of vitamin supplements. In
fact, to many people the word "vitamin" itself is synonymous with

the little pills or capsules we take to ensure we're getting the required amount of vitamins. We've got it all backwards.

If there is one thing I'd like you to take out of all the biochemistry in this chapter, it is this: nature has given us the ideal delivery system for getting all the vitamins (and minerals, for that matter) we will ever need. That system is called <u>whole foods</u>. Vitamin supplements are intended to be just that - supplements for when we fail to eat the right foods. Use your food as your primary vitamin source and you should need few if any pills. There are some other very significant reasons for avoiding pills and capsules, which we'll be discussing in later chapters.

Summary of Vitamin Sources / Daily Values

Vitamin	Source	3-Day Target
Vitamin A	Liver, green plants	4,000-5,000 IU
Vitamin B-1	Beans, nuts, eggs	1.5 mg
Vitamin B-2	Grains, nuts, eggs	1.7 mg
Vitamin B-3	Grains, eggs, beans	19 mg
Vitamin B-6	Poultry, fish, beans, nuts	2 mg
Vitamin B-12	Intestinal bacteria, meat	2 ug
Folate	Green vegetables, orange juice	200 ug
Panthothenate	Mushrooms, broccoli	6 mg
Biotin	Peanut butter, cheese	30 ug
Vitamin C	Citrus, fruits, greens	60 mg
Vitamin D	Milk, cheese	5-10 ug (200-400 IU)
Vitamin E	Nuts, oils	30 IU
Vitamin K	Green vegetables	60-80 ug

Vitamins
To Wage War

1) **Try to get as much of your vitamin requirements as possible from whole foods rather than supplements.** Use the list above to identify and select foods that are high in vitamins.

2) If you take multi-vitamin supplements, buy from major manufacturers, and use in moderation. One multi-vitamin every 3 - 4 days should be plenty if you're eating right.

3) Never buy vitamins that do not have expiration dates stamped on the package. Discard your old vitamins.

4) Do not take antioxidant supplements (Vitamin E/Vitamin C/beta-carotene) every day. A carrot a day gives you a satisfactory dose of Beta-carotene (5 IU) and is a better source than a pill.

5) Do not exceed daily targets for B vitamins. Neurological problems can result from excessive doses. If you take "stress" formula vitamins (B/C combinations) with large amounts of B vitamins, cut the tablets in half to moderate your dosage.

6) Two vitamins for which you can occasionally exceed target values are Vitamin C and Vitamin E. Vitamin C can be taken up to 250 milligrams every other day. 200 milligrams per day of Vitamin E may prevent certain diseases.

Chapter 11
MINERALS

Vitamins are large and complex molecules; minerals are small atoms, though every bit as important. Minerals serve as cofactors in many enzymatic reactions. Phosphorus, for example is needed to break down sugars. Minerals are necessary for cells to grow and reproduce; zinc is a cofactor in an enzymatic reaction involving DNA. In many ways, the essence of a mineral is its electrical charge; minerals contribute these charges or use them to bond in certain ways.

Though essential, minerals are micronutrients, needed only in small amounts. It's generally not necessary to take mineral supplements, since you get plenty from your food under most circumstances. All minerals are toxic if you get too much.

CALCIUM

Calcium enters your cells from the bloodstream and serves many functions. Nerve impulse transmission, cellular adhesion, muscle excitement, muscle contraction and blood coagulation are a few of the most important functions of calcium.

The calcium level in your blood is always the same. Blood calcium is not directly influenced by diet, but tissue levels can vary. If the blood level ever changes, serious consequences and even death can result. Hyper/hypocalcemia can result in obvious tremors, tetany (from a potentially fatal calcium deficiency), and rigor in your muscles.

The calcium in your bones is stored from dietary intake through about the age of 25. From this point onward, your cells struggle to maintain bone density and avoid Osteoporosis, a bone depletion that can make you susceptible to serious fractures. Adult calcium intake is used to replace lost calcium and maintain your storage levels. The calcium-to-potassium ratio in your bone is about two to one.

Bone is a dynamic and complex material made mostly of two structural components; a strong matrix and groups of cells. The matrix, hydroxyapatite, is a porous molecule that includes calcium, phosphorus, oxygen and hydrogen. The three main groups of bone cells are called osteoblasts, osteoclasts, and osteocytes. Osteoblasts form the hydroxyapatite and other support structures. Osteoclasts break down bone for resorption when calcium supplies are low. Osteocysts are dead osteoblasts surrounded by the matrix. They release their calcium to the blood as needed.

There is an annual turnover of 2 to 4 percent of the extracellular matrix. It provides a continual opportunity for you to renew your good health and eat right. If you are not eating foods that are good for you, substitutions can be made for calcium in your bone matrix. Substitutions for calcium can be made by magnesium, sodium, fluorine, carbonate, citrate, strontium, and lead. These substitutions create varying levels of harm to the bone structure. This doesn't mean you should avoid foods with magnesium, for example. In fact, a low magnesium level can precipitate a low calcium level (Hypomagnesemia = Hypocalcemia). It does, however, allow us to consider replacing excessive carbonated beverages or foods containing citrate with high-calcium foods.

Incidentally, while your teeth are a bone structure, they are made of a compound like hydroxyapatite that does not break down as easily and does not help regulate blood calcium levels.

Calcium has also been found to be important in regulating blood pressure. Pregnant women sometimes experience a rise in blood pressure which can be corrected with an increase in calcium consumption. During pregnancy, 1200 mg/day is recommended

Deficiency Symptoms
Osteoporosis is the most publicized condition related to calcium deficiency, although blood coagulation problems and muscle cramps are other potentially serious consequences.

Risk Factors/Protective Factors For Osteoporosis

High Risk Factors:	Female Thin Alcoholic Clumsy	White Old Steroid use Cigarette smoking
Moderate Risk Factors:	Low Calcium Level Thyroid Problems Vitamin D Deficient Sedentary Lifestyle	Early Menopause Antacid Use (non-Calcium) Type I Diabetes
Possible Risk Factors:	Family History Alcohol Use High Fiber Diet	Caffeine Use High Protein Diet
Protective Factors:	Exercise Obesity Dark Skin	Calcium Intake Estrogen Children

Common Fractures In Osteoporosis

Thoracic or lumbar vertebrae
Wrist
Hip
Compression of vertebral column

Recommended Dietary Allowance

The USRDA for calcium is 800 milligrams daily. More is needed for pregnant women (1200 mg/day) or young teens who are still building their bone calcium stores.

Toxicity

Quantities up to 2500 milligrams per day will not seriously harm the average person, provided you don't do it all the time and provided that your sources are natural foods and not supplements.

Adverse effects associated with excess calcium intake can include the following:

Constipation -	Calcium salts harden feces
Kidney stones -	Can seriously damage kidneys
Upset mineral balance -	Too much calcium and there can be iron and zinc depletion

Calcium Homeostasis (Regulation)

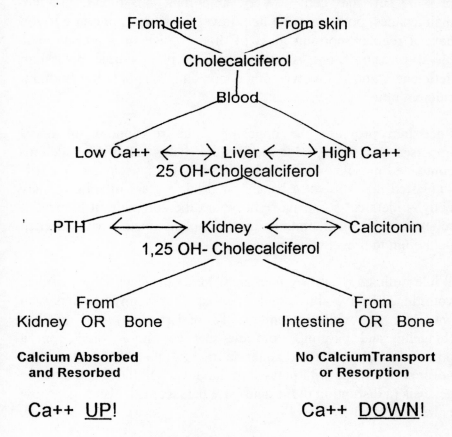

From diet   From skin

Cholecalciferol

Blood

Low Ca++ ⟷ Liver ⟷ High Ca++
25 OH-Cholecalciferol

PTH ⟷ Kidney ⟷ Calcitonin
1,25 OH- Cholecalciferol

From
Kidney   OR   Bone

From
Intestine   OR   Bone

**Calcium Absorbed
and Resorbed**

**No CalciumTransport
or Resorption**

Ca++ <u>UP!</u>   Ca++ <u>DOWN!</u>

Ca++ = Calcium
Cholecalciferol / 1,25-OH / 25 OH =Forms of Vitamin D

POTASSIUM

Potassium is a catalyst for energy reactions. It also helps maintain pressure in the cell. Very important in blood pressure maintenance, potassium can help lower your blood pressure if you have a regular morning glass of orange juice or a banana. The blood pressure story is more complex than simple potassium deficiency, and it involves other ions and the potassium/sodium/calcium ratio.

Potassium provides the opposing force to Sodium in nerve impulses and, along with Magnesium, helps relax the Calcium-contracted muscle. This is why, if you have muscle cramps, it is suggested that you eat a banana or drink a glass of milk. Many bodybuilders eat a banana right before the competition because it relieves their dehydration and supplies them with needed potassium to prevent cramping.

While deficiency is rare, potassium loss can occur with diarrhea, vomiting, laxative abuse, and bulemia. One of my students who was both anorexic (pathologically underweight) and bulimic (bingeing and purging), told me that he almost died from a potassium-induced heart abnormality and that his doctors had never seen anyone with potassium that low! Diuretics and diabetic acidosis (a disruption in the acid-base balance) can also trigger low potassium levels.

Symptoms of deficiency are also seen in starvation situations and in "Kwashiorkor" or protein deficiency. In destitute countries, mothers with several children can see these deficiencies in their older children. "Kwashiorkor" is an African phrase meaning "the spirit that takes over the first child after the second child is born". Once a child stops nursing, it often has very little nourishment and suffers the symptoms of malnutrition. One of the characteristics of Kwashiorkor is the **flag sign**. A horizontal strip across the middle of the hair is colorless indicating this deficiency.

Symptoms of Potassium Deficiency

Muscle weakness
Lowered intestinal tonus
Heart abnormalities
Flag sign
General fatigue

Recommended Dietary Allowance
2 - 6 grams per day is the USRDA. This translates to about 1.4 grams per 1000 calories of food.

Toxicity
Toxicity results in Hyperkalemia where the excretion is less than the intake. This can occur in hospitals where too much is given through a feeding mechanism, or if you take too many supplements. 18 grams per day is often a fatal dose.

PHOSPHORUS

Phosphorus is a macro-mineral, meaning it is found in large amounts in the body. In fact, you have 11 - 13 grams of phosphorus per kilogram (2.3 lbs.) of body weight! Phosphorus is extremely metabolically important! Most of it is found in our skeleton or bone. The calcium to phosphorus ratio in bone is 2:1. If you look at the Calcium Homeostasis chart, you'll see the way that phosphorus is regulated also. It works in concert with Vitamin D and calcium regulation. Phosphorous is most absorbable in the form of phosphate. The kidney is the primary site for regulation, not the intestines.

Phosphorus functions in bone mineralization, collagen formation, ATP (energy) production, and acid-base balance in blood plasma, phospholipids, DNA, and enzymes.

Deficiency Symptoms
Very few people have phosphorus deficiencies, because this mineral is readily available in many foods. However, pre-term infants can be low in phosphorus, and they may need a supplement to assist in bone development. An adult phosphorus deficiency, called Hypophosphatemia, can result from malabsorption, diabetes, phosphate binders in food, alcoholism, urinary loss, starvation, and eating disorders. (When helping a starving person, it is best to rehydrate them slowly first, then start nutrient supplementation. If rapid repletion occurs, the system of the starving person can go into shock, or acute Hypophosphatemia can result.)

Phosphate binders in food include phytates, fiber, and antacids. Heavy antacid use over long periods of time can deplete phosphorus, resulting in bone loss, breakdown of body tissues, weakness, and bone pain. In diabetes, as in alcoholism, acidosis and acidic conditions result in great urinary loss of Phosphorus. Other symptoms of Hypophosphatemia are lethargy (no ATP is made - See the Carbohydrates chapter), confusion, red blood cell deformity, insulin resistance and glucose intolerance, seizures, and coma.

Recommended Dietary Allowance
800 milligrams per day; 1200 milligrams for pregnant women.

Toxicity
There is a concern that we may get too much phosphate, in the form of soda or pop. If you drink a lot of soda, you are getting quite a lot of phosphate. Thirty percent of the recommended daily intake of phosphorus can be obtained from a can or two of soda. This may be a concern in young children or post-menopausal women whose calcium intake is low. Poor development and all the symptoms that accompany calcium deficiency can result. For post-menopausal woman, osteoporosis becomes a possibility.

There is also a lot of phosphorus in meat and animal products. If you eat a lot of meat, you may be calcium deficient (as well as overweight, have high cholesterol, etc.)

SODIUM

Sodium is the subject of much publicity, mostly negative. My own opinion is that much of this concern is unfounded. Sodium helps maintain osmotic pressure in the cell, and functions as a basic ion to keep blood pH-neutral. Sodium also helps regulate nerve impulses.

Deficiency Symptoms
Weakness, nausea, and ultimately death can result if you get little or no sodium. There's very little chance of this happening in the U.S. today, because so many of the foods we consume are loaded with sodium. Sodium is depleted as we perspire during competitive sports or heavy workouts. We normally lose less than a gram per day unless we participate in one of these events. In Addison's disease, there can be tremendous losses of sodium because the hormone aldosterone is lacking. Aldosterone (in the adrenal gland) regulates sodium levels. Chronic diarrhea, renal

disease, serious illness like cholera, and accidental injury all precipitate sodium loss.

Recommended Dietary Allowance
It has been stated by informed scientists both that there is no RDA for sodium, and that the RDA is 1000 milligrams (or 1 gram) per day. I tend to favor the latter opinion. It is human nature to jump to conclusions and brand one nutrient as a bad actor. We need sodium to live. It is actually very unwise to limit sodium during pregnancy, for example, even if there is edema.

Toxicity
Sodium has been branded as bad for people worried about high blood pressure. It is only bad for you if you are sodium-sensitive, which many people are not. If you are not sodium-sensitive, there is probably little reason to worry excessively about sodium intake, unless it is more than 4 - 5 grams per day. Remember that it is not just the level of sodium in your blood, but the interactions between all the pressure-regulating cations like potassium and calcium that counts.

One way to offset a high sodium level is to make sure you get enough potassium along with your sodium. This can be accomplished by consuming more fruit, orange juice and a banana per day. (A good idea anyway!) Calcium also works; a glass of skim milk or yogurt will do the trick.

MAGNESIUM

Magnesium is widely distributed in all green vegetables and some animal products. Magnesium is found in the center of every molecule of chlorophyll, which is the molecule that gives green plants their green color. Magnesium is important in many body functions including enzyme reactions for Glycolysis, ATP production, the TCA cycle (see the chapter on Carbohydrates), and neuromuscular transmission.

Magnesium is somewhat antagonistic to calcium in that they share similar electrical charge and functions. The relationship is so close that hypomagnesemia (low concentrations of magnesium) leads to hypocalcemia (low concentrations of calcium). Another good reason to eat your vegetables!

Magnesium is the ion of choice when formulating solid soap products because it combines with fatty acids in such a way as to keep them in a solid form in a bar of soap.

Good sources of magnesium include cocoa (!), spinach, nuts, whole grains, molasses, soybeans, and clams. These sources have almost 50 milligrams of magnesium in every 100 grams (about a quarter pound) of food.

Deficiency Symptoms
The availability of magnesium in the body is inhibited by several factors including malnutrition, solubility, alcoholism, diarrhea, and low protein intake. Vitamin B-6 is always found with magnesium as a cofactor. The combination has a sedative action. There are occasionally magnesium deficiencies in the U.S., especially among alcoholics. Fat malabsorption is one of the ways Magnesium deficiency manifests itself.

The symptoms are remarkably similar to B vitamin deficiencies, partly because the population often having a deficiency is the same population with B vitamin deficiencies; namely, alcoholics. The other reason for similarities is that both B vitamins and magnesium affect the central nervous system (CNS) and neuromuscular sites.

Symptoms of Magnesium Deficiency	
Memory lapses	Concentration problems
Apathy	Depression
Confusion	Hallucinations
Paranoia	Numbness
Cramps	Tremors
Muscle weakness	Nystigmas
Ataxia	

Recommended Dietary Allowance

The RDA for magnesium is 300 - 450 milligrams per day. The diet of an average adult supplies enough magnesium.

Toxicity

Magnesium toxicity is rare. In healthy people, the kidneys process and excrete excess magnesium. Toxicity may occur in individuals with kidney failure or malfunction, due to reduced elimination in urine.

SILICON

The most abundant mineral on earth, silicon acts very much like carbon and can be found both in free form and bound to other elements. Silicates are found in foods as additives (anti-caking agents). The silanolate ester and mucopolysaccharide forms are more absorbable. Fiber, molybdenum, magnesium, and fluorine all affect absorption of silicon.

Silicon works to form crosslinks between collagen, elastin and mucopolysaccharides to make them strong and resilient. Active in connective tissue, silicon helps in the synthesis of bone and collagen through the enzyme, prolyl hydroxylase. Silicon is very important in the building of young bone tissue. It is layered early during the calcification of bone and calcium later replaces it.

Symptoms of Silicon Deficiency	
Poor joints	Weak bones
Badly formed skull	Reduced growth
Bone has less water	Cartilage separates from bone

Toxicity
None really, but there may be immune implications, such as with leaking breast implants and the onset of autoimmune disease and breakdown of tissues. Too much magnesium trisilicate (antacid) is not a good idea.

MANGANESE

Manganese comes in two active chemical states (as do most of the divalent cations). These states are Mn^{2+} and Mn^{3+}. It can become attached to magnesium metalloenzymes like Superoxide dismutase or Pyruvate carboxylase. There is a high concentration of manganese in your bone, liver, and pituitary gland (about 3 micrograms per gram). The concentration is low in muscle and plasma (0.4 - 0.8 micrograms per gram). These concentrations remain relatively stable throughout life.

Only about 3% of our dietary manganese is absorbed. That which is absorbed is changed in the liver from Mn++ to Mn+++. Transported by a protein called transferrin, excess Mn++ is excreted in the bile.

Symptoms of Manganese Deficiency

Bones/skull - short, thick, bowing
Cartilage - defective due to lack of Glycosyl transferase
Joints - enlarged
Muscles - Gastrocnemius slips occasionally
Reproductive - pregnancy maintenance
Glucose Tolerance - impaired
Neonatal Ataxia - otolith (inner ear) underdeveloped;
Low coordination with head retraction occurs in utero

Recommended Dietary Allowance

There is none, but the Safe and Adequate Intake (SAI) level is 3 - 5 milligrams per day. The average American diet contains 2.9 milligrams per day. A consumption of 0.7 milligrams per day is considered deficient.

Toxicity

Too much manganese can result in growth depression. Airborne contaminants (for miners) create Parkinsonian syndrome (L-Dopa can help). Too much manganese reduces hemoglobin synthesis and iron absorption by competing with iron for sites on the transport protein transferrin. One gram (1000 milligrams) is a toxic dose.

ZINC

Zinc is vitally important to many body functions including cell growth, sexual maturation, night vision and immune repairs.

Taste and Zinc - Zinc plays a role in taste and appetite. Hypogeusia (lowered ability to taste) and Dysgeusia (inability to taste) can be caused by low zinc levels. So if you have an elderly parent or grandparent who cannot taste as well as they once did, have them try zinc lozenges (COLD-EEZE™ has 13 milligrams of zinc gluconate per tablet) for a day or two. Remember, though, zinc is hard on an empty stomach.

<u>Vitamin A and Zinc</u> - Zinc is involved in Vitamin A and vision functions as well. In a zinc deficient situation, you can't mobilize Vitamin A from its storage in your liver. Vitamin A is then unavailable to the body for conversion of Retinol to Retinoic Acid (forms of Vitamin A). There may be another reason to eat your carrots after all. You get zinc along with a theoretical double-dose of proVitamin A when you eat a carrot. Otherwise you'd need to remind yourself about both zinc and Vitamin A all the time.

<u>Sex and Zinc</u> - Lack of zinc can be associated with reproductive failure, low fertility, and teratogenesis (birth defects). Low zinc levels are often found in individuals with dwarfism or hypogonadism.

<u>In The Cell</u> - There are over 200 enzymes in the body that require zinc as a catalyst to function properly! In this way, zinc affects all of the major biochemical pathways. Cell division and replication of DNA both require zinc as a cofactor. Without it, problems such as the teratogenicity mentioned above and irregular cell replication can result. There are base pair changes (see Chapter 4), odd polypeptides, irregular transcription and lots of other DNA problems as well. Zinc levels in the nucleus of your cells are a direct reflection of your zinc intake, unlike most other nutrients.

<u>In The Immune System</u> - Your immune system needs zinc for speed of response to infection, immune cell proliferation, to make IgG, and to enhance the cell-mediated response to invaders.

Symptoms of Zinc Deficiency

Skin disorders
Sexual dysfunction
Vision problems
Immune dysfunction

Recommended Dietary Allowance

12 milligrams per day is the RDA for zinc. If you eat a lot of meat, you're probably not zinc deficient. More than the daily dose can be toxic.

Toxicity

Zinc intake of 18 - 25 milligrams every day can inhibit copper functions in your body. Levels of 100 - 200 milligrams per day causes disorders like hypocupremia, neutropenia, microcytosis and immune impairments. This level can also cause a drop in your HDL (the "Good" cholesterol) level. Two grams (2000 milligrams) creates acute toxicity and can be fatal.

SELENIUM

Selenium may be protective against heart attack and stroke. It functions as an antioxidant in your cells. It works in concert with Vitamin E and gluthathione peroxidase (an antioxidant enzyme) to prevent liver damage, and indications point to a protective effect against several types of cancer (including colorectal, esophageal, lung and prostate cancer).

Deficiency Symptoms
There appears to be little chance of selenium deficiency in the U.S. Most of us get about 100 micrograms every day. To avoid deficiency, eat whole grains, mushrooms, asparagus and brazil nuts (which have just about a daily dose per nut).

Recommended Dietary Allowance
An intake of 50 - 200 micrograms per day is considered safe and adequate for adults, but 60 micrograms is the most you should probably take per day.

Toxicity
Selenium can be very toxic in high doses. In one well-publicized case in 1984, eleven people were poisoned by an accidentally high dose created by a manufacturer of supplements. These individuals lost hair and fingernails, vomited, and had general malaise. It has also been suggested that, while protective against some cancers, Selenium could enhance the growth of others like Hodgkin's disease and leukemia.

IRON

Necessary for the creation of functional hemoglobin, iron helps hemoglobin hold on to oxygen molecules that we take in when we breathe.

We need Iron, Vitamin B-12, and Folate to make a red blood cell. Any dietary deficiencies might create problems in the production of blood cells. Binding compounds (ligators) in the intestine also affect absorption. Dry beans, a major world protein source, can interfere with absorption of iron. Heme iron (animal derived) can enhance absorption of non-heme iron. Hypoxia (resulting in low iron content) regulates erythropoesis (the making of red blood cells). Iron is stored in the liver, spleen, and bone marrow. It can be found bound to hemoglobin (in your red blood cells) and transferrin (a transport protein) in the bloodstream. In muscle it is bound to myoglobin (muscle protein).

The bioavailability of iron is affected by many factors:

Factors Affecting The Bioavailability of Iron

Negative	Positive
Fiber	Acidity
Phytic Acid	Vitamin C
Non-heme Fe+	Heme Fe+
Tannins	Certain amino acids
Caffeine	Increased Need
Repeated Pregnancy	
Geophagia	
GI problems	
Low Vitamin B-12 / Folate	

Iron carries oxygen (O_2), Carbon dioxide (CO_2), and, unfortunately other compounds. These other compounds include the poisonous carbon monoxide (CO) gas that is trapped in stationary cars or in poorly ventilated rooms using space heaters. A famous tennis star recently found this out the hard way, and basically suffocated when his red blood cells carried carbon monoxide instead of oxygen. Iron is also involved in hemopoesis (blood cell creation), enzyme activity, immune system function, and learning and behavior (low iron = poor learning). It is involved with the cytochromes of the oxidative phosphorylation system and low iron can affect work, performance, and exercise capabilities.

Deficiency Symptoms
We have a two- to three-day supply of old iron that is lost when the cells slough off. New iron is needed at least that often. Iron taken in pill form is less bioavailable than in the form of whole foods. Intestinal helminthiasis can cause deficiency as can gastrointestinal problems. Deficiency symptoms can include weakness, headache, dyspnea (shortness of breath upon exertion), angina, claudication (leg pain), and paleness in conjuctiva, fingernails and skin. Fatigue and miscarriage are sometimes a result of iron deficiency. Sports anemia or hemoglobinurea can result after a long competition, especially in long distance runners or in high impact exercises. Capillary breaks are a result of the pounding of the body. Amenorrhea is a result of excessive high impact sports as well.

Recommended Dietary Allowance
The RDA is 15 milligrams per day for average adults. Children need a bit less, pregnant women a bit more. To treat deficiency, a physician may administer as much as 200 - 240 milligrams daily for up to 6 months. This is only in very severe cases.

Toxicity
Hemosiderosis can create excess storage of iron and in hemochromatosis, a rare genetic disorder, excess iron causes liver damage and eventually death. If children find and eat adult vitamins, they can die as a result of the high iron concentration.

CHROMIUM

Chromium functions in two major capacities, glucose tolerance and lipid metabolism. In the late 1950's, a Dr. Mertz labeled chromium "the Glucose Tolerance factor". Many nutritionists were reluctant to accept this designation and the debate continues today. In spite of this questioning, there are several facts to consider.   Chromium is a factor in the creation of a good antioxidant, glutathione. This helps regulate carbohydrates in the cell.

Chromium also helps regulate lipid metabolism. A low chromium level leads to atherosclerosis and high hyperlipidemia (some lipids rise, others are lowered).

Deficiency Symptoms
A major symptom of chromium deficiency is the raising of insulin and abnormal glucose tolerance which results in a diabetic-like state. At risk for chromium deficiency are those on TPN (Total parenteral nutrition - feeding tubes), pregnant women, the elderly, those with a food allergy (whose food needs to be purified), and those with malnutrition.

Recommended Dietary Allowance
The RDA for chromium is 0.09 milligrams per day.

Toxicity
While relatively safe at RDA levels, chromium can be toxic in very large amounts. To avoid the interference of chromium with other cationic minerals (like iron), stick to the RDA or lower.

SUMMARY

The table below summarizes the important types, sources and recommended intakes for minerals. As in the case of the vitamin values in Chapter 10, the listed target values are for normal, healthy adults.

My recommendation for mineral intake is the same as that for vitamins: go easy on pills. You are always better off getting your minerals from a balanced diet rich in whole foods than by taking

supplements.   If you use supplements, do so sparingly, and only
on the advice of a qualified professional.

Summary of Mineral Sources and Daily Values		
Mineral	**Food Sources**	**RDA/3-Day Target**
Chromium	Orange juice, vegetable oils, prunes, peas	0.09 mg
Selenium	Garlic, squash, lean pork	0.12 mg
Iodine	Shellfish, salt	0.15 mg
Molybdenum	Carrots, tomatoes, squash	0.25 mg
Fluoride	Tea, wheat germ, almonds	2.5 mg
Copper	Nuts, oysters, whole grains	2.5 mg
Manganese	Pineapple, berries, tea	3.5 mg
Zinc	Whole grains, meats, seeds	12 mg
Iron	Molasses, meat, raisins	15 mg
Magnesium	Dark green veggies, nuts	350 mg
Calcium	Dairy, dark green veggies	800 mg
Phosphorus	Dairy, nuts, soda, fish	800 mg
Sodium	Salted foods	1500 mg
Chloride	Fish, eggs, salt	1800 mg
Potassium	Fruit, veggies, lean meats	3000 mg

Minerals
To Wage War

1) **Try to get as much of your mineral requirement as possible from whole foods rather than supplements.** Use the list above to identify and select foods that are high in minerals.

2) **Drink an 8-ounce glass of skim milk, or eat one cup of yogurt each day.** This will help lower blood pressure and reduce your risk of osteoporosis.

3) **Eat a brazil nut** every so often to ensure you get enough selenium.

4) **Eat bananas** to provide potassium and help keep blood pressure down.

5) **Iron stores are important.** To keep yours up, try lean meat or black strap molasses.

6) **Eat your veggies!** They contain significant quantities of virtually all essential minerals.

Chapter 12
WATER

Our bodies are composed mostly of water, yet we often ignore water as one of the most important nutrients. All body fluids are fundamentally water; urine, blood, saliva, lymph, perspiration and digestive juices.

Given the importance of water in our nutrition, it's surprising how little thought most of us give to the quantity and quality of the water we drink. This chapter should give you some food (drink?) for thought regarding the largest component of our diet.

How much water should you drink?

Approximately eight 8-ounce glasses of liquid per day, or 64 ounces, is a good amount for an average 150-pound body. If you weigh considerably more or less than this or if you exercise heavily, you should adjust your intake accordingly. This intake can come from water or other fluids. Just remember that along with water, other drinks may contain less desirable components like excessive sugar, artificial color/flavor or caffeine. Eight glasses of water are healthy; eight cups of coffee or cans of cola are probably not a good idea. Water from fresh fruit and vegetables also counts toward our daily liquid target.

If you suspect you are not drinking enough water, increase your water consumption gradually until you feel you've reached the correct amount for you. Don't try to drown your cells by increasing intake all of a sudden. Also, drink water gradually over the course of a day rather than all at once. Too many individuals are robbing themselves of electrolytes and needed nutrients by diluting themselves with water.

Water In Your Food / Water Activity

Water is found in your food in different concentrations. Produce is about 90-96% water. Crackers are much lower in water content. This content is crucial to the taste, breakdown due to bacteria or molds, and texture of your food. This water content is referred to as A_w or **Water Activity** by food scientists and nutritionists. Water activity is one measure used to determine whether certain microbes will grow in different foods.

Knowing what foods can harbor what bacteria also allows you to figure out the source of foodborne illnesses. In the chapter on Food Safety (Chapter 13) there is a guide to selected microbes describing the foods they contaminate according to water content.

Our Water Sources

Our water comes from varied sources such as wells and municipal utilities. We also get our water from the store in bottles; perhaps an expensive way to have reassurance that isn't absolutely guaranteed. Where your water comes from gives you clues as to what's in it - both good and bad.

Municipal Water
Did you know that most municipal water is recycled? In other words, we are all not drinking from that pristine lake nearby; no, we're drinking the recycled waste water (sewage, wash water, bath water) of our neighbors and residents in nearby communities! There isn't enough fresh, new water to keep up with our increasing

demand, so much of our water isn't "fresh". I was shocked when I first found this out many years ago.

Bacteria in this recycled water is the reason that so much chlorine (bleach) is added. It is one of the only ways to kill most bacteria without harming pipes (though chlorine does corrode them over time). Other antibacterial substances are added to water as well.

Well Water

Many homes have their own water wells or are supplied with water pumped from municipal wells. Water from these wells often harbors other man-made or naturally occurring compounds. If you have your own well, you owe it to yourself and your family to have the water tested periodically.

Chemical contaminants from industrial and agricultural sources can seep into the ground over time and enter the groundwater supply. These contaminants can travel for long distances underground, so just because you don't live next to a farm or a factory doesn't mean your well water is necessarily clean.

Radon, a naturally-occurring radioactive material, can build up in groundwater in certain areas and become airborne when water is aerated at your tap or shower head. You run the risk of exposure when you drink the water or breathe the airborne radon into your lungs. Radon is now believed to be the second leading cause of lung cancer in the U.S., behind cigarette smoking.

Bottled Water

Fearing the quality of our tap water, many of us buy bottled water for drinking. We are under an amazing illusion that all bottled water comes from primordial underground springs in pristine locations, untouched by man except for the tube that carries it out to those plastic containers for us.

In fact, the vast majority of bottled water does not come from naturally-occurring springs; most of it is bottled tap water from all over the place. And getting water from a natural source is no guarantee of quality either, as our discussion on well water pointed out.

Bottlers use numerous techniques to purify water. One method, reverse osmosis, forces tap water against a concentration gradient through a membrane. This membrane is usually very fine and can remove much of the possible contamination contained in the **RECYCLED** water that is used! In other words, you may be drinking bottled water from your own municipal water supply (or from Love Canal, for that matter).

The back of the label always says where the company is located or where the water is bottled. At least it used to. I just found a brand of bottled water in my local supermarket that has no location written anywhere on the bottle. And it doesn't say how the water was "created"... In spite of the fact that you are drinking "used" water, reverse osmosis works very well at removing most contaminants. Assuming that the filter is changed often. And those filters are expensive! That's motivation enough for water companies to sleaze the most time out of one of their water filters! Call them and ask exactly how your water is produced; at almost $1.00/gallon, don't you have a right to know?

If you want to find out if your bottled water company is a member of the organization which holds them to strict testing rules, call:

International Bottled Water Association (IBWA)
Alexandria, VA
(800) WATER 11

Have Your Water Analyzed

No, not by the person who comes to sell you water-softening equipment, but by a testing lab like the one below. The water softening people are only performing a few tests, which are generally designed to make you purchase a water softener. Use major labs - that you have to pay - for analysis if you want accurate results.

National Testing Laboratories, Inc.
6151 Wilson Mills Road
Cleveland, OH 44143
(800) 458-3330

The costs vary, but are never exorbitant (usually under $100) and it might be worth your trouble.

If you're wondering what you can do if the water has chemicals in it that you don't want - there are a variety of home filtration systems to get rid of the contaminants. A valuable secret I learned from the water-softening people is that you can use a simple total-house carbon filtration system to remove radon from your water. The ones that the radon companies will try to sell you are very expensive and little more than a simple charged carbon filter, so it is a way to save money while cleaning your water of radon. It must be replaced or recharged every year or so, however.

What Could Be In Your Water?

In a word - anything. Most water contaminants are the result of environmental pollution, but some, like metals and radon, may also occur naturally. You'll note that some of these metals are among the essential minerals we discussed in the last chapter, but the

quantities and chemical forms of these metals may render them
unhealthy, even toxic.

What's In Your Water?

Metals:

Arsenic	Iron	Selenium
Barium	Lead	Silver
Cadmium	Manganese	Sodium
Chromium	Mercury	Zinc
Copper	Nickel	

Pesticides:

Alachlor	Heptachlor	Silvex
Aldrin	Hexachlorobenzene	Simazine
Atrazine	Hexachloropentadiene	Toxaphene
Chlordane	Lindane	Trifluralin
Dichloran	Methoxychlor	2,4-D
Dieldrin	PCBs	
Endrin	Pentachloronitrobenzene	

Organic Compounds (this is only a sampling):

Chloroform	1,3-Dichloropropane
Bromodichloromethane	2,2-Dichloropropane
Dibromochloromethane	1,1-Dichloropropane
Bromoform	Ethylbenzene

Organisms:

Algae	Protozoans
Bacteria	Viruses
Fungi (molds & yeasts)	

Particulate matter in your water needs to be removed along with unwanted chemicals. The Drinking Water Book gives the example of a 5 micron filter; it will trap all particles that are larger than 5 microns. If your water is very dirty, you will need a larger filter like a 50-100 micron filter.

Size of Typical Particles Found In Your Water*

Viruses	0.01-0.1	microns
Smoke	0.05-1.0	microns
Dust	0.1-5.0	microns
Bacteria	0.1-40	microns
Pollen	10-100	microns
Hair	20-300	microns
Dirt	20-600	microns
Fog	50-150	microns
Sand	100-5000	microns

1 micron = one millionth of a meter

*(*Adapted From The Drinking Water Book)*

If you'd like more information on water, I highly recommend that you read **"The Drinking Water Book" by Colin Ingram** (Ten Speed Press, 1995), which has far more information than can be given here.

Water
To Wage War

1. Never drink distilled water from plastic containers.
Minerals present in regular water can prevent the water in plastic jugs from absorbing too many of the harmful plastic compounds from the container. Distilled water has these removed, so the protective effect is lost.

2. Try to get most of your water from glass containers.
Glass containers are generally "inert"; that is, they do not contribute any chemicals to the liquids held inside them.

3. Use potassium or calcium salt to soften your water..
Potassium salt instead of conventional sodium salt can provide a nutritional benefit. Ask for K-Life at your hardware store.

4. Avoid drinking chlorinated water.
This will help you avoid the carcinogenic Trihalomethanes (THMs) which may be created when chlorine encounters organic compounds.

5. Have your tap water tested.
Water picks up contaminants within piping, so always test at the final exit point (your tap). Testing should be done by an independent company (one that does not sell water treatment equipment).

6. Treat your own water if needed.
Here are a few tips. **Boil** water to kill bacteria. **Stir** water to remove volatile compounds, or **let water sit,** open, for a few minutes. **Let the water run** for three minutes to flush out water which has accumulated lead and heavy metals.

THE FRONT LINE

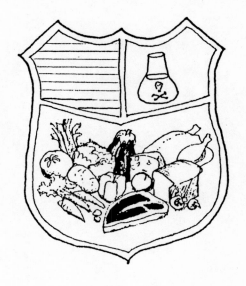

Chapter 13
FOOD SAFETY

Several old Monty Python routines addressed our fears about food and dining out. The next few lines from one of the routines are part of a conversation between an "average" couple about what is offered for dessert.

Wife:	"We've got rat cake, rat pudding, rat sorbet and strawberry tart."
Husband:	"Strawberry tart?"
Wife:	"Well it has got some rat in it..."
Husband:	"How much?"
Wife:	"Three, rather a lot really..."
Husband:	"I'll have a slice without so much rat in it."

Reprinted courtesy of Python (Monty) Pictures, Ltd.

It always amazes me how we feel we must compromise our own health and safety for conformity. Consumers often feel helpless when dining out. This chapter is meant to arm you with information so that you don't need to eat "the slice without so much rat in it".

Monitoring Your Local Food Establishments

Have you ever had an episode where you vomited or had diarrhea or gas hours or days after eating out? If so, there's a 90% chance it was from something you ate. Food infection is one of the most under-reported illnesses, largely because people are never sure what caused it or where they encountered it. Here are some guidelines for you to use to avoid food illness AND be able to identify the source on your own. I hope you will use this information to keep your local restaurants and food establishments on their proverbial toes when it comes to cleanliness and food preparation.

Filth in Food

According to the Fundamentals of Microanalytical Entomology (A.R. Olsen et al, 1996), filth in food can be broken down into five all-encompassing categories:

I. Filth from vectors of food borne disease
Examples include:

Bat hair	Rodent excrement	Feather filth
Human hair	Beetles	Ants
Mites		

II. General filth that is non-pathogenic
Examples include:

Dermestid beetles   Dust mites

III. Live infestations or other outrageous adulterants
Examples include:

Earwigs   Spiders   Insect Fragments

IV. Filth from insects stored in the product
Examples include:

Flour weevils

V. Incidental filth
Examples include:

Soil   Dust   Glass shards

Typical Foods That Cause Food Illness

Meat dishes / Gravy - Undercooked
E. coli .

Escherichia coli (*E. coli*) is a Gram-negative intestinal bacteria that causes serious food-borne illness by producing a toxin (called Verotoxin). It likes warm, moist environments in which it can multiply. There are four basic categories: ETEC; EIEC; EPEC; and EHEC. While all four types produce a toxin, the most dangerous is EHEC (Entero Hemorrhagic Escherichia Coli). This causes hemorrhagic colitis. The result is sudden, severe, crampy pain and bloody, watery diarrhea accompanied by renal (kidney) or colonic (colon) lesions. There is seldom a fever, but if you get this kind of *E. coli* infection, death could result.

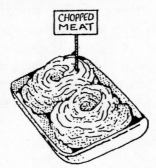

Beef or pork that is undercooked can harbor *E. coli* bacteria. You are likely to have more of this bacteria in ground meat than steaks or chops because in ground meat there is the opportunity to have the surface bacteria mixed thoroughly throughout the meat. Timing is a major factor. Any amount of time at room temperature encourages the bacteria to grow. You are also safer with chops or steaks because the bacteria is only (usually) on the surface and gets heated during cooking to a temperature sufficient to kill it. Not in rare steak or steak tartare.

You're taking your life in your hands with undercooked meat! Think it'll never happen to you? I'll bet you think that "they" (whoever "they" are...) have taken precautions against this so you can safely eat out. Guess again.

The few instances recently at major fast food restaurants have killed people! They didn't just go home with a tummy ache, they died! These incidents were "traced" to the process of slaughter, where it was surmised that during the part of the process where the organs are torn away from the meat, the intestine was perforated. In the U.S., the government responded with changes to the process so that no intestinally contaminated meat would reach the market. But who's minding the store?

We also get meat from other countries who don't have to abide by our regulations. And as with all new regulations, enforcement is a big issue and there are not enough inspectors to go around. Up until two or so years ago the meat inspectors in this country certified meat by just looking at it! Unbelievable! I know I've never seen a bacterium with my naked eye...Have you?

So now that the process has changed, you feel reasonably comfortable. Well, don't. If your butcher didn't wash well enough after using the bathroom, he could harbor this bacterium on his hands and work it into your meat! We have it in our intestines too! Your mother-in-law could put it in her meatballs! A baby whose diaper you've just changed could be the unwitting cause of food illness. The only answer is to follow the cleanliness regimen outlined later or avoid the type of meat described above.

Poor Hudson Foods, the beef company in the midwest that had to shut down because of *E. coli* contamination. They unfairly took the brunt of consumer wrath for the entire meat industry. We are now under the illusion that with them gone, all of our meat is safe.

Unfortunately all meat producers are very similar and this will happen again someday.

Meat - Cooked
Trichinella spiralis
Insufficiently cooked pork can contain trichina, or juvenile worms. These worms mature in the walls of the intestines of the hosts, both human and other animals, and create havoc and pain. The young worms go into the blood vessels and head for the muscles of the chest, ribs, eye, tongue and jaw. This migration of up to one million tiny worms causes muscle pain, fever, anemia, and if serious enough, respiratory failure and death. People are often misdiagnosed with intestinal troubles.

Once in the muscle the worms grow to about 1 millimeter and encyst (enclosing themselves in a protective package). The adult worms do not usually harm the host; they either die or look for a new host that ingests the flesh they sit in. If the flesh of an infected animal is eaten by another uninfected animal (such as humans), this new animal becomes infected.

How do pigs get this? Is it checked for in our food supply? An answer is found in these paragraphs from "Animals Without Backbones" (R. Buchsbaum, 1987).

"Pigs obtain worms by eating the flesh of other animals, sometimes rats but usually fragments of other slaughtered pigs included in uncooked garbage. In the body, pigs go through the same history as described for human infection."

*"At the present time the U.S. government does not inspect pork for the occurrence of encysted trichina worms, since such inspection requires microscopic examination and light infections could be readily overlooked anyway. **Inadequate inspection is worse than none, because it gives a false sense of security to the consumer.** The absolute prevention of trichinosis lies with the consumer, who has only to cook all pork and pork sausages thoroughly."*

If large pieces are to be roasted, it is especially important to determine that heat has penetrated to the center; large public barbecue picnics are often a source of epidemic trichinosis. An ounce of heavily infected pork sausage may contain 100,000 encysted worms. If half of these are females, and each gives rise to 1,500 juveniles, the host would have to cope with 1.5 million juveniles, enough to cause death. All market animals are parasitized in some way or other, and it is understood that consumers will prepare food in such a way as to safeguard themselves against infection."

Beef
Mad Cow Disease
Mad Cow Disease is caused not by a virus, but by a prion, a much smaller infectious protein particle. Called both Scrapie (in sheep) and Mad Cow Disease (in cattle), it causes sheep and cattle to exhibit unusual behaviors such as rubbing themselves continually up against rough surfaces until they have open bloody wounds. It is very difficult to detect in food, as are viruses. *Post mortem* analyses of the brains of infected people, sheep, and cows reveal the unusual progression of the disease.

Even more troubling is the ability of the prion to resist attempts to destroy it. Prions appear to remain infectious even after 30 minutes of boiling, two months of freezing, two years of drying, and exposure to formaldehyde, chloroform, carbolic acid, and ultraviolet light. The fact that prions can resist UV light set at a wavelength to destroy DNA indicates that we may have something in our food supply which is virtually indestructible.

One aspect of this that interests me is the strong relationship with Creutzfeldt-Jakob syndrome, where patients lose their minds as well as their physical abilities. I personally know of two heavy meat-consuming Creutzfeldt-Jakob sufferers who died recently. Richard Rhodes' "Deadly Feasts" (1997) gives some insight into the elusive nature of this horrifying disease.

In this book, Dr. Rhodes examined an intriguingly similar disease among New Guinean cannibals called Kuru. The disease, which produced symptoms such as uncontrollable giggling, dramatic personality changes, shivering and twitching, was called "Laughing" disease by the natives. It was shown that this debilitation started with small pieces of filamentous protein (possibly linked to some sort of nucleic acid trigger) that created amyloid deposits (plaques) in the body and brain of infected patients. Rhodes called it "the strangest thing in biology", and cited Dr. Igor Klatzo (a neuropathologist with the National Institutes of Health) who said that "the widespread involvement of various brain structures does not fit into any of the known hereditary degenerative patterns."

The discovery of prions, and the realization that they are not like viruses, fungi, bacteria, or any other known infective particle, is truly frightening. Equally disturbing is how easily prions can get into the food supply, taking advantage of our modern methods of beef production. Here's how.

Dairy cows are raised to produce milk. Farmers keep them doing that by "freshening" them or forcing them to calve three or four times during their stay on the farm. This works for a while, but like all mammals, they have a reproductive limit and after four years or so, milk production slows and they are sent away. TO BECOME HAMBURGER!!! That's right! Much of our hamburger is made from DAIRY COWS! Beef cattle provide the larger cuts of meat. If you erroneously think that we are carnivores, you might be thinking, "So, meat is meat, right? What's the big deal?"

To keep their milk production up, dairy cows are given drugs and are fed diets rich in protein supplements. Beef cattle are given the same protein supplements later in the process and eat mostly grain to begin with. This high-protein supplement given to dairy cows, according to Richard Rhodes and others, has traditionally been mostly made of ground up DOWNER CATTLE! Downer cattle are cattle with brain cancer, other cancers, neuromuscular deformities (that cause them to fall down, hence the name) or the amyloid plaques of Altzheimers and Mad Cow Disease. This has been the cheap, easy way for farmers to get feed.

This practice has resulted in death for several British citizens from what was originally diagnosed as Creutzfeldt-Jakob syndrome. It was later diagnosed as Mad Cow Disease. This is the hamburger connection. Even the New Guinea cannibals discovered that you definitely are what you eat. Dead meat.

While herds of cattle and sheep are being destroyed in Britain and around the world, this does not mean that this infective agent is eliminated. Prions are amazingly elusive. Future routes of transmission might include eating pig flesh, having organs transplanted from animals, contact with surgical instruments that appear to have been sterilized, dusting your roses with bone meal, taking hormone injections or eating lunch at any meat-driven fast food restaurant.

While not prevalent in this country, Mad Cow Disease is probably now in the U.S. food supply and has up to a ten year incubation period. The USDA and FDA have instituted new regulations to prevent this, but total enforcement is nearly impossible. Don't let the government tell you not to worry. Let's stop making cannibals out of our livestock and do things the right way, not the cheap way. As Rhodes says, "...sometimes meat bites back..."

To Make Beef Safer:

Your only 100% effective alternative is to avoid beef altogether. If that prospect is more than you can handle, here are some ways to minimize your risk.

Protecting against *E coli*:
Avoid all ground beef/hamburger; stick to prime cuts
If you do eat hamburger, cook it thoroughly
Wash all surfaces immediately after working with raw beef
Use a good antimicrobial agent

Protecting against Mad Cow Disease:
Eat domestically produced beef
(U.S. livestock are somewhat safer than European herds)

Find out what your cattle ate - inquire at your market or call the supplier.
(Specifically check if offal is part of the food source.)

Note: Food preparation techniques appear to have no effect on the prion that causes Mad Cow Disease!

Chicken / Eggs and Egg dishes
Salmonella typhimurium
Salmonella typhi
Salmonella enteriditis
Salmonella is a type of Gram-negative bacteria found in the intestines that is the number one cause of food infection. It produces diarrhea, cramps, mild fever (if some of the heat-sensitive toxin remains) and (rarely) vomiting. It also likes warm, moist environments in order to reproduce and lukewarm eggs are a perfect place.

There was a big controversy in New Jersey recently when the
powers that be banned Hollandaise sauce, Caesar salad, eggs over
easy, and all other dishes that use raw eggs. They were attempting
to protect the public from itself. It was a good idea, but it is hard
to legislate food preferences. "Damn the torpedoes, I'm having my
Hollandaise sauce" was the hue and cry from the hoi polloi and
thus a law was shot down.

Not every egg carries *Salmonella,* but a good portion do. Several
years ago, it was believed that avoiding cracked eggs was
sufficient to avoid the bacterium. More recent tests have revealed
Salmonella in the ovaries of many hens, where it can be inserted
into many eggs that reach the market. You can get *Salmonella*
other ways, but raw eggs is one of the best ways.

To Make Eggs Safer:

Use only fresh eggs
Do not use cracked eggs
Make sure your supermarket has all eggs at a good, cold temperature
Always refrigerate your eggs
Throw out eggs that have translucent spots or lines
Never wash eggs unless you use them immediately
Do not use if the yolk is weak or collapses when opened
Do not use if the white is cloudy or yellow
Do not use if there is blood inside

Chicken meat is also a good source of *Salmonella,* especially if it is
undercooked. Chickens and other poultry are often copraphagic
(they eat their own feces) possibly due to underfeeding of proper
nutrients by poultry farmers. Whatever the reason, the meat of
chickens and their surrounding environment contains lots of
Salmonella.

> **To Make Chicken Safer:**
>
> Wash all surfaces immediately after working with raw chicken
> Use a good antimicrobial agent
> Store only 3 - 6 months in freezer, then throw out if not consumed
> Store only days in refrigerator
> Keep cold at all times
> Thaw in refrigerator, not under water or on counter
> Rinse with clean water before preparing for cooking
> Cook until no pink is present in the center of the meat

Around the turn of the century, there was a heavy-set cook named Mary. She worked in a restaurant in New York City where she both cooked and served the food. People that frequented her establishment began coming down with typhoid fever. Few reported it, and several cases were missed because the people died before anyone could question them. After some time, the wheels of the health inspector's mind began turning and he centered on this restaurant, but since no one was sick who worked there and there were no real standards of cleanliness to enforce, the case was dropped.

The case picked up after more people who ate at this restaurant acquired typhoid, and began to focus on Typhoid Mary. If people ate there on the days that she was off, they were fine. But if they ate when she cooked, they likely acquired the disease. So she was asked not to work in food establishments anymore. She refused and was locked up in isolation. One fine day when allowed out to exercise, she escaped. Months later, following a typhoid outbreak in upstate New York, she was found again, and she lived out her days in confinement. And the public was protected for a short time

in the Star Trek sense. "The needs of the many outweigh the needs
of the few".

Milk and Cream / Soft cheese / Eggs

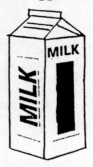

Listeria monocytogenes
Listeria is a common, underreported bacteria with an unusual
habit. It flourishes in the COLD! It is found in slaughterhouses,
dirt, animal feed, and dairy products such as those mentioned
above.

There was a recent incident in the Southwest where homemade
Mexican flavored soft cheese was the culprit. They had used raw
or unpasturized milk to make the cheese. *Listeria* causes
miscarriages, psychoses, encephalitis and sometimes death. It is
largely found in animal products.

Dairy Products
Staphlyococcus aureus
A common indigenous (lives in some people all the time)
microorganism, *Staph* may not always cause disease in the host,
but can still be deadly for others. It, like any other microorganism,
can mutate over time to become virulent or infective.

A flight from Hong Kong to San Francisco touched down in
Hawaii and picked up breakfast. Ham and cheese omelettes with
bagel slices were waiting on the tarmac - since the day before. In

fact, they had been sitting in the heat for 14 hours before being loaded on the plane. All of the passengers were served starting about 9:15. The crew was served last. The crew had a special breakfast of pancakes and sausage that had been delivered just before take-off. As they were enjoying their breakfast, one of the male crew members, who had wolfed his breakfast down, went back to eat any leftover passenger breakfasts. There were several. He ate two of them.

Within an hour all hell broke loose. *Staph* is often referred to as the <u>double bucket organism</u>, because it's one of the few microbes that carries a bonus; you get sick at both ends. Imagine 345 passengers, one crew member, 3 bathrooms and everyone has both vomiting AND diarrhea! My professor used to refer to it as "The Vomit Comet". Not a pretty picture, is it?

There was one unusual fatality in this story. The omelettes had been made in the kitchen of a Japanese chef with a boil on his thumb that he'd accidentally lanced while cooking. Testing revealed that the *Staph* in his boil was the *Staph* that made the passengers sick. The chef, upon discovery of this fact, committed suicide in his kitchen with his sword, in the traditional Japanese manner.

To Make Dairy Products Safer:

Buy only pasteurized products
Don't try to make your own cheese or yogurt unless you really know how
Use only major manufacturers who must adhere to FDA standards
Call the manufacturers and ask about their sources of milk/cream
Keep very cold; it will help a lot for other organisms, a little for *Listeria*
Use well before manufacturer's suggested Sell-By or Use-By date

Salad Vegetables
Salad provides the most incredible variety of microorganisms of any food, because it passes through so many different aspects of processing. Let's examine lettuce as an example. As it grows, it can be fertilized with animal waste that may contain microbes of concern. It can then be picked by a migrant worker equipped with inadequate sanitary facilities, who relieves himself in the field and cannot wash his hands before he picks your lettuce. He might be ill or have a bacterium or virus that is also rubbed on your lettuce; and both infectious elements can remain viable for a lot longer than you think.

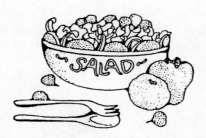

Next the packager, washer, and store employee or cook's assistant all touch the lettuce without gloves, leaving their own personal microbes for you to consume. And if it's left at a salad bar, I can almost guarantee from working on the Board of Health that the sneeze guard is not sufficient and is there for show only. Don't forget the guy who works part-time who puts the salad out and may or may not be clean. And that's just the people who touch your <u>lettuce</u>. How about the people who did the carrots? The machinery is often contaminated with filth and bacteria too. And of course, you do not heat or cook salad to kill the bacteria.

Ascaris lumbricoides
Worms! Poorly washed salad vegetables or strawberries can harbor ascarids, or parasitic nematodes. Nematodes come in many

sizes from microscopic to visible with the naked eye, but *Ascaris lumbricoides* nematodes which inhabit the intestines of both humans and animals can be up to 20 inches (40+ centimeters) long! The eggs pass out in the feces and can infect other animals through the fecal-oral route. These worms are endemic in some areas of Thailand and China, and can also be found in other countries due to demographic shifts.

When the eggs hatch in the body, the worms take a trip through your body, boring through lung tissue into the bronchii where they ascend to the throat and are swallowed. They leave the intestine, having dined on partly digested food, and burrow into the blood vessels. They resist digestion, but can die spontaneously in about a year. It is the migration that does the host the greatest damage. With up to 5000 worms per infection, they can do much damage. Oral antiworming medication sends them running through body organs like the liver; they have even come up the esophagus and out the victim's nose!

To Make Produce safer:

Purchase from a reputable, clean grocer
Wash and soak all produce, then wash again
Inquire about the company that supplies the store
Call the produce company; ask probing questions - you have a right to know!
When you can cook it - Do!
Use Mayonnaise or Acidic Dressing

Rice / Potatoes
Clostridia botulinum
Few people think of rice or potatoes as vectors for deadly disease. If we're unsure of a restaurant, we might say, "I'll just eat the rice" thinking we'll be safe. This might work, or it could backfire big time.

I always enjoyed the stories my professors used to tell about microbial disease in foods, and I regularly share them with my students today. Here are two more tales of woe; these involve *Clostridia botulinum*.

A middle-aged man on a flight from Paris to New York had pre-selected a special in-flight dinner. He was the only passenger on the flight to have this meal which consisted of lettuce, rice, green beans, almonds and mandarin orange segments covered in a sweet dressing. His dinner was brought first and he did what we all do before we eat: he sniffed the food. He then tasted a bit of it. He asked the passenger next to him if it didn't smell funny to him. The passenger, upon sniffing it, replied "Whew! That smells awful!" The man in our story then pridefully decided it was fine and ate it. By the end of the ride he was paralyzed from the neck down, <u>permanently</u>. That's what botulism and botulinum toxin can do to you. The moral? Use all of your senses and do what they tell you to do! If it smells funny, don't eat it!

While botulism is known as the dented can organism in the supermarkets - and is the reason you should never buy dented or swollen cans - it can live in any anaerobic (oxygen-deprived) atmosphere. It is a soil organism and is primarily associated with produce. Any food grown in soil has the possibility of carrying the organism. But it's not unusual to be complacent about it because we associate food-borne illness with fatty or proteinaceous foods like creams and meats, not produce.

One of the biggest potential botulism culprits is chili. Cooked in large pots, it cools slowly allowing the organism to grow in the warm gooey substrate. It is often reheated several times. The *Clostridia botulinum* or *Clostridia perfringens* is happy in this anaerobic environment because all of the oxygen has been cooked out of the thick mixture. Where does the microbe come from? The beans or onions. With heavy soups, it is best to thoroughly clean vegetables before cooking, and when cooling, separate the mixture into smaller portions.

Botulism from *Clostridia botulinum* and illness from the related, but less dangerous, *Clostridia perfringens* can result from simple acts such as putting your shoes on kitchen surfaces. This allows soil-borne organisms to take up residence on your counters. Not to mention other people's expectorations, squirrel dung, old pieces of gum, dead skin and anything else you might collect on the bottom of your shoes. Floor things (brooms, shoes, paper bags from the supermarket, etc.) need to remain at floor level to insure that your working area is relatively free of soil-borne germs. Which brings me to my second botulism story.

A 60-year-old woman had just heated up a commercial pot pie (for 45 minutes) for dinner when her husband burst in with fast food for the two of them. A nice gesture. She couldn't refuse him, turned the oven off and set the pie on the back of an unrefrigerated shelf. They ate the burgers, watched TV and went to bed. It wasn't until three days later, around dinner time, that she noticed the pot pie. Not wishing to expend the effort to cook, and since the pot pie had had some oven time, she ate it. Paralysis and death were the result.

Peanut Butter / Corn
Aflatoxin
I always recommend Skippy brand peanut butter to my classes. Why? Because years before other peanut butter manufacturers bothered, Skippy manufacturers recognized and did something about one of the most dangerous toxins we know, Aflatoxin.

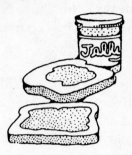

Aspergillis flavus is the organism that creates aflatoxin if given the right conditions for growth. You won't immediately get sick as a result of ingestion, but you are exposing yourself to serious cancer potential. Responsible manufacturers still need to get on this issue and respond. A plant pathologist colleague of my father's up at Cornell alerted me many years ago to the necessity of using care with this toxin.

Aflatoxin creates serious problems because it is chemically very similar to a DNA base. This means it can substitute for components of your normal DNA and thus integrate itself into your DNA whenever new DNA is being made. And that's every day! This integration can cause strange things to happen within your cells as a result. These strange goings on often precipitate cancer.

How Can We Prevent Aflatoxin From Getting In Our Food?

1) Find responsible manufacturers.
2) Ask questions about corn and peanut products.
3) Ask if producers use the black light Kojoic acid test.
4) Ask what percentage of their corn or peanuts are removed from the stream of food product.
5) Ask HOW they remove aflatoxin from the food. The answer should be that the whole peanut or ear of corn, etc. is discarded.
6) Use only nuts or corn that are a typical color; avoid dark versions of these foods.

Strawberries / Raspberries

Cyclospora

Cyclospora, a microbe that usually isn't associated with large outbreaks of disease, has been creating problems in fresh and frozen raspberries and strawberries lately. Food scientists and microbiologists are wondering where it came from in the processing of the berries. Look no more. It more than likely came from someone's dirty hands.

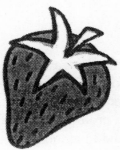

We like to try and find any machine, stream of water, or other non-human source of contamination to deflect away from the obvious. But the truth is that most contamination is the result of poor personal hygiene on the part of a food worker or sloppy food handling after contamination by a food worker. By continually ignoring the obvious we put our population at risk. All of these complex and contrived HACCP (see next section) and Irradiation plans, while obscuring the view of the general public, will never really help. Education and enforcement are the only answers.

Pseudomonas, a fairly ubiquitous bacterium, was recently found in contaminated strawberries. Want a rude surprise? It probably was put there on purpose by the grower! What I'm trying to say is that growers of strawberries and any other appropriate fruits actually apply *Pseudomonas* in a wet spray to their crops. You see, the bacteria are genetically altered (Biotechnology rears its ugly head!) to prevent susceptibility to freezing temperatures, so when they're coating strawberries with the slime, farmers can preserve their crops longer. This doesn't address the possibility of them staying on the fruit after it's harvested or mutating into infective strains that threaten our health. This goes on all over the country without our consent or knowledge. Also, when making a bacterial slurry for spraying it is easy to contaminate it with other harmful bacteria who enjoy the same medium or food. It's worth thinking about when buying berries.

Sushi / Raw fish
For intestinal excitement, eat raw fish! Ah, there are so many possibilities, I don't know where to begin. Let's talk about microfilaria, or microscopic worms. Responsible for terrible diseases, pain and death around the world, these little worms were seldom seen or mentioned in association with food in the U.S. But sushi and sashimi have changed all that.

The Chinese Liver Fluke, *Clonorchis sinensis*, is common in China, Korea, Japan, and other parts of Southeast Asia. In certain regions of China, greater than 75 percent of the population is afflicted. The biggest problem with microscopic and even larger worms is the cercariae or cysts that hide in the muscle tissue that we consume. The young flukes, freed by digestive juices from their capsule, now burrow into the bile ducts of the liver. Serious liver disease, anemia, and even predisposition to liver cancer are the result.

We seldom think that consuming rare or undercooked muscle tissue exposes us to anything serious. We believe this so strongly that some of us actually eat raw fish! A dangerous prospect even if the restaurant's a good one or you know the chef!

Supermarket Fish / Cancer

Go into the seafood section of one or two local supermarkets and look for fish with cancer. I guarantee you'll find several. Look for an irregular white or grey mass with tiny blood vessels in it. You can usually see these in the fish muscle like filets or salmon steak.

Sometimes the fish with cancer are prominently displayed. Having seen one on a regular visit to the fish section one day, I informed the fish man and the manager. Both of them looked at me like I was crazy. The fish man said, "That's not cancer; that's just extra fat or something. We see those all the time." As you might suspect I left totally reassured that our food supply was safe. (Not!)

Raw or Undercooked Fish / Hepatitis A

Hepatitis A is a serious viral pathogen that can find its way into your seafood (and other foods). It can lead to liver dysfunction and predispose you to liver cancer. It is most often found in seafood caught in polluted water contaminated with sewage. The oral-fecal route is the easiest way to transmit the virus. This also means that it is possible to get this from a kitchen worker who has hepatitis.

No one wants to discriminate against anyone with communicable diseases. But when it comes to food preparation and service I have to ask: WHY NOT? Isn't the health of the many patrons of a food establishment worth moving a sick worker to garbage pick-up or parking lot duty? It is so hard today to say or do anything that might be offensive to anyone that we risk people's health right and left.

We need to use clean gloves in ALL food preparation. We need relatively healthy individuals in hair nets, gloves and masks to do this preparation if we are to be safe. You know there are more germ precautions taken with computer chips than will ever be taken with your food!

Why do restaurants allow sick people to continue to work with food? I have three possible answers to this question.

1) In an unethical world, it's considered O.K. by some restaurant owners for sick people to work out of sight, because patrons who get sick can't PROVE that it was the restaurant. Ah, but you CAN prove it! If you suspect your food made you sick, you can ask the Board of Health to take samples of what you ate. The problem with hepatitis, though, is that it doesn't initially have severe symptoms and there is a 30 day incubation before you might see jaundice or feel weak, etc.

2) The other, more legitimate reason restaurants allow sick workers to make your food is that you can't always tell if someone is sick by looking at them. And God forbid you should look at someone's appearance, listen to them coughing, consider them unclean, and refuse to let them work. The hue and cry about discrimination would lift the roof!

3) Economic considerations govern the third reason you will find sick workers at food establishments. Food service workers are hard to find. The pay is relatively low, the turnover is great, and few people want to make it their life's work. I know. I worked at most of the major fast food chains in high school and at a couple of restaurants in college.

Norwalk Virus

One of my favorite horror stories about a food virus that was not transmitted by food involves Norwalk virus, a parvovirus which is found in a variety of foods and produces vomiting, diarrhea and abdominal pain.

In 1971, a professor at a Midwest college asked two individuals to volunteer for a scientific experiment. I have to assume that they were doing this for brownie points because they were behind in his class or something. They both agreed. He explained that he was testing Norwalk virus to learn about the course of infection. He then told them, I think, about a fellow volunteer currently in the hospital with this virus and implied a sense of urgency to this project. And in a move so unethical audiences gasp everytime I talk about it, he inoculated these students with culture from the patient in the hospital. With a milkshake of mashed feces and water that he watched them drink! He then counted and measured their bouts with fever, diarrhea and vomiting. Makes you wonder...

It would probably be no comfort to these individuals to know that the data collected was probably useless anyway because of the small human sample, the odd route of inoculation, and several other unscientific elements.

Why New Food Pathogens Emerge

Changes in Eating Habits
We now eat more fresh, exotic and unusual fare. We are also more reliant on convenience foods.

Increased Awareness
Databases are able to locate and report even small numbers of cases.

Demographics
Our populations are shifting and as a result, more sensitive groups occur.

Changes in Primary Food Production
We are now on a global scale of food production. Controls are much more difficult. The example I always give my students is to look at a typical New York restaurant breakfast (See chart on the following page) of scrambled eggs, bacon, wheat toast, coffee or tea, orange juice and fresh fruit. Where could these ingredients and products be produced?

Changes in Food Processing
Vacuum packaging, modified atmosphere packaging, chilling and microwaving foods add a measure of irregularity to microbial growth.

Handling and Preparation
In the home there are hazards we may be unaware of like the microbes on the countertop or in the refrigerator or freezer.

Changes in Microbes
The same reason that you need a flu shot every year is the reason that old bacteria re-emerge as a virulent strain and new viruses, fungi, and bacteria are found to cause disease: mutation. It can change a harmless microbe into a dangerous one and a harmful one into non-disease causing. Mutation is an ever-present force that governs our lives.

Typical New York Breakfast

Scrambled Eggs
Eggs from farm in Vermont
Milk from Pennsylvania
Butter from Wisconsin
Salt from the Midwest / Pepper from South America
Scrambled in New York

Bacon
Pigs born in United Kingdom, raised on Canadian farm
Pigs slaughtered in New Jersey
Bacon shipped to New York

Wheat Toast
Wheat grown in Iowa, ground and shipped to Ohio
Dough conditioner from New Jersey firm added
Baked in Connecticut
Shipped to New York

Coffee/Tea
Coffee grown in Sri Lanka / Tea grown in Colorado
Water from Westchester, New York
Sugar from Puerto Rico
Milk from Wisconsin
Made in New York City

Orange Juice
Oranges grown, processed and dried to powder in Florida
Flavorant chemicals from California added
Shipped to New Jersey and rehydrated with local water
Consumed in New York City

Fresh Fruit
Bananas from Ecuador
Grapes from Chili
Grapefruit from Florida
Apples from New Zealand

The Hazard Analysis Critical Control Plan (HACCP)

HACCP is the most current method being used to assess potential microbial harm from a given food source. It is a systematic approach designed with the manufacturer in mind. HACCP infers that all that is needed to ensure food safety is to find one or two serious "critical control points" and adjust them. It reduces the number of times and amount of product a manufacturer has to test. It is designed to virtually eliminate end-product testing. It does provide some regulatory control as well.

To assess hazards, the HACCP plan looks at food Growth (plants in the field, animals in their pens), Harvest and Killing Procedures, Processing, Distribution and Manufacture, and finally Preparation and Use. Pretty comprehensive? Well, it tries to be. But it still doesn't address, in a large enough way, the fact that undereducated food workers are the primary cause of contamination. Nor does it address the fact that all food workers (in every type of food service!) should be required to take an introductory Microbiology course. A course like my Microbiology course! That would put the fear of God into them. I can't count the number of times I've heard, "Really, Dr. Walters...You can get it that way?!" or "That's gross; I never knew that..." We need to have an educated population or there will always be some unfortunate, innocent individuals who pay for this ignorance with their lives.

HAACP Principles

Find microbial contamination
Stop growth
Get microbes out
Keep them out

Locating Control Points in Food Manufacturing

1. Review/evaluate process flow chart - locate areas of concern
2. Maintain good records and review them regularly
3. Provide consumers with product recall information:
   Toll free #
   Batch # on package
   Good distribution
   Verification system
4. Label packages with important consumer information
   e.g., "Keep Frozen"
5. Review Time/Temperature information on the product
6. Provide employees with adequate education

This plan focuses not on the organism, but on its introduction into the food production process. Let's follow the making of homemade chili in the flow diagram on the next page. Look at each step and notice how contamination can occur.

Chili Production: Biggest Problems (in descending order)

Poor cooling of cooked food
12 or more hours between preparation and eating
Infected persons handling food
Inadequate reheating
Inadequate hold hot temperature
Raw food contamination
Unsafe food sources
Improper cleaning of utensils
Cross contamination from raw to cooked food
Inadequate cooking of food

Chili Contamination Profile

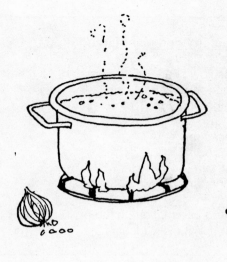

Cooking kills most bacteria except *Clostridia botulinum*

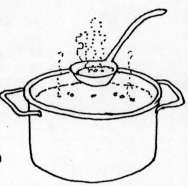

Serving introduces more human microbes to the chili

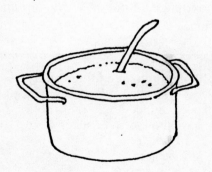

Holding at warming or room temperature allows rampant microbial growth!

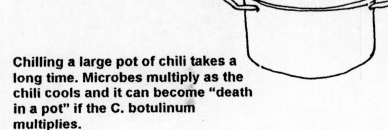

Chilling a large pot of chili takes a long time. Microbes multiply as the chili cools and it can become "death in a pot" if the C. botulinum multiplies.

Identifying Your Foodborne Illness

Water Activity

Look at how moist and unsalty your prepared food is. Heavy salt or heavy sugar concentrations can be antimicrobial in some cases. A water activity of 0.95, for example, means that the food is very moist, and probably lower in salt or sugar than another food. All the organisms below can be found in **all of the foods** at the same water activity. So any 0.95 A_w organism can contaminate any 0.95 listed food.

Food	Type Of Organism	Water Activity
Fresh vegetables	*Pseudomonas*	(0.95)
Meat, Fish	*Escherichia*	40% sugar
Cooked sausages	*Shigella*	7 % salt
Canned foods	Hepatitis	
Milk	*Clostridia*	
Breads	*Listeria*	
Cheese, ham	*Clostridia*	(0.90+)
Fruit juice	*Salmonella*	55% sugar
Applesauce	Molds, yeasts	12 % salt
Dry cheese	*Micrococcus*	(0.80+)
Ferm. sausage	*Vibrio*	65% sugar
Cakes	*Candida*	15% salt
Margarine	*Lactobacillus*	
Fruit juice / syrup	*Penicillium*	
Sweet cond. milk	*Staphylococcus*	
	Saccharomyces	
Jam, marshmallows	*Aspergillus*	(0.70+)
Oats, nuts	Halophilic bacteria	
Dried fruit	Xerophilic Molds	

*Adapted from Food Chemistry (Fennema, 1985)

Temperature Requirements
Different bacteria thrive at different temperatures. If you know the general conditions under which your food was consumed, you can use the table below to narrow the possible microbial candidates.

Type of Bacteria/Examples		Temperature Information
Thermophile	*Bacillus thermophilus*	Likes warm temperatures; 60 degrees Celcius (140°F). Refrigeration limits growth of thermophiles.
Psychrophile	*Pseudomonas* *Aeromonas* *Lactobacillus*	Grows in refrigeration. Sometimes freezing. Need to thoroughly heat foods.
Mesophile	*Staphylococcus aureus*	Lives in warm-blooded animals like ourselves. These are typical pathogenic bacteria. They prefer body temperature; 37 degrees Celcius (98°F). Cook foods well. Use high acid foods.
Halophiles	*Halobacter*	Prefers extreme environments; high salt and high heat. Can exist in very dry conditions. Not usually pathogenic.

Symptoms of Food Illness
Look carefully at the symptoms you get and when they arrive. An early infection might likely be a bacterium like *Staph*, while one that hits you several days after you ate something questionable could be *Salmonella* or hepatitis. *Clostridia* infections are usually very clear and easy to self-diagnose.

• *Listeria* - Miscarriage and headache are two possible results of ingesting the bacterium *Listeria monocytogenes*, which causes the disease Listeriosis. Homemade cheeses, yogurt and milk products can harbor growing colonies of *Listeria*.

• *Staphylococcus* - *Staphylococcus aureus* or *epidermiditis* can be commonly found growing on people's hands. Bacteria that isn't pathogenic to you might kill your best friend! Be careful! Watch out for warm, proteinaceous foods like meats or cream dishes. Staph infections generally result in vomiting and diarrhea (a double bucket organism). Note that they begin as early as 1 hour after eating and last a short time (several more hours)!

• *Streptococcus* - Poor Jim Henson (the beloved Muppeteer) felt he was coming down with the flu and ignored the symptoms of weakness, vomiting and malaise. He went to bed early, but died within days. Strep A, also sometimes known as the flesh-eating bacteria, can consume you in a very short time. Responsible for Strep throat and Toxic Shock Syndrome as well, it can have dire consequences. Be aware of injuries that redden and grow warmer long after they've been iced or heated.

• Hepatitis - Responsible for much undiagnosed misery around the world, hepatitis has a very long incubation period, up to

30+ days. Its symptoms are jaundice (yellowing around the eyes and other thin skin) and fatigue. If you feel that a restaurant might not be up to your cleanliness standards, don't eat there! If you must eat sushi, be sure and drink alcohol with it; it is one of the few possible ways to prevent an infection.

- *Clostridia perfringens* - This species of *Clostridia* is often called "The buffet organism" because it grows in food left out warming. It creates lots of gas and gas pains, but is often over in a day or two, without dire consequences. *Clostridia* species are brought into your home on your raw and frozen vegetables, dry beans and on your feet. It is a soil-borne organism, which is why I suggest that you never put floor items on your countertops or food preparation surfaces.

- *Clostridia botulinum* - This bacterium produces a deadly toxin that can kill you in a very short time. The toxin does not have a smell that you would recognize, but a food such as rice or canned string beans will have a strong off-odor if contaminated with *Clostridia botulinum* (See botulism story). Symptoms include intolerance to exercise, weakness, dizziness, breathing difficulty, double vision. Within only a few hours after infection you can be permanently paralyzed! If you experience any of these symptoms after eating out or eating home-canned food, run to the nearest emergency room!

- *Salmonella* - *Salmonella* infection is very common. It is more than likely what you get when you come home with diarrhea from eating out, or after you eat raw cookie dough, etc. It is only serious to the elderly, immune compromised and the very young. It is a nasty inconvenience for the rest of us. *Salmonella* appears anywhere from 12-36 hours after you eat contaminated food. Symptoms include diarrhea and occasional vomiting.

Food Safety
To Wage War

1) Insist on gloves for all food handling personnel. It's your right!

2) Conduct your own cleanliness inspection and grade each food establishment.

3) Boycott supermarkets and restaurants that don't meet your cleanliness standards.

4) Speak to the manager everywhere you go that appears to be unclean.

5) Write a letter to the editor of your local paper about filthy eating or serving places.

6) Write to the corporate headquarters about your local branch supermarket or restaurant.

7) Call the local Board of Health, hope they're not overburdened, and ask them to check out your findings.

8) Get hold of a consumer reporter at a local or national radio or TV station and describe what you've seen.

9) If you are a food worker, or know a food worker, use literature (such as excerpts from this chapter) to alert the owners or fellow employees of health issues in the food establishment.

10) Throw out any suspect or old food; your health is worth the few extra dollars!

Chapter 14
FOODS: TOXIC AND
CANCER-CAUSING

Foods Are Chemicals

A food is a group of known and unknown chemical compounds that is modified by various factors: pesticides, contaminants, processing, and storage. Later in the process, a food may be further changed by the addition of food additives, more contaminants and the preparation procedure. In your body, food is further modified by digestion, absorption and metabolism.

One of my professors used to say, "An effective chemical is a poison". His rationale was that a chemical that was effective was also toxic at some level. How do we decide what is toxic in your food and what is safe?

Determining the Toxicity of Food

In a May 1996 article in the Journal of the American Medical Association (JAMA), an interesting statement was made: **"Food is the largest antigenic challenge facing your immune system."** We seldom consider that food, which keeps us alive, may also help do us in. It is an important consideration. How is this antigenic challenge presented to us on a daily basis? In what form does it come? Is it in all foods? Are all foods equally affected?

There's no need to panic unnecessarily here. There are simple ways to prevent exposure to too many toxic compounds. The first is to understand what makes a compound toxic.

To be "toxic", a chemical must be capable of doing harm. It must also have three aspects:

A Toxic Substance Has

A chemical or physical agent
A biological response from an affected system
A harmful effect

There are many factors affecting the toxic nature of a substance. Its chemical, physical (size and shape), storage, and stability characteristics are the first, basic aspects of its toxicity. But no chemical stands alone for long. Does it dissolve in biological fluids? Are there additional agents such as adjuvants (liquor in cough syrup), extractants (an example is hexane in decaffeinated beverages), coloring agents, binding agents, and surfactants?

The Dose Makes The Poison

This is a common phrase in toxicology, because even water is toxic to your system if you get to much of it. There was a case of a grossly overweight man who decided to just drink water instead of eating in order to lose weight. He died within two weeks from loss of electrolytes and nutrients due to the excess water. Is that what we mean by toxic? Not usually, but it can be made to fit the definition.

The dose is relevant, though, especially when you consider the site of administration. If you regularly work with motor oil and spill half a can on your hands, you'll be O.K. If that same half a can goes down into a water system, you have contaminated thousands of gallons. That water is no longer fit to drink. If you drink that water and expose yourself to the toxins in the oil, there are much more serious consequences than exposing your intact skin.

In addition to the dose and route of entry, we must also consider the rate, the duration, the frequency of exposure, the time and the site of administration to complete our toxicological picture.

Limonene is considered a poison. It is regularly added to the "fresh-squeezed-not-from-concentrate" orange juice of a major company (discussed in the Tricks section at the end of the book). Limonene also has antioxidant properties. These antioxidant properties are negated by the way it is inserted into the juice. Not just negated, but turned into something far more heinous. Now the American Cancer Society recently endorsed orange juice as a good anticancer substance. I have to assume that the American Cancer Society doesn't realize about the backlash of antioxidants (See Antioxidant Secret #1) and the poisonous nature of the limonene that is added to much of our orange juice, or they wouldn't have endorsed packaged orange juice. The company that produces the orange juice rationalizes, I suppose, that the average person doesn't drink that much orange juice in a lifetime anyway. Risk assessment skips toxicity and cancer-causing capability, and moves right on to usage and quantities. A consumer myself, I want to know if there is ANY RISK, and then I'll make my own usage decision, thank-you.

Alcohol is a toxic substance absorbed by the stomach. We instinctively know this and do our own detoxifying of alcohol. We know that if you eat foods before drinking, especially fatty ones, they will coat your stomach and prevent alcohol absorption. That is why it is suggested that you eat before going out drinking.

Factors Affecting Toxicity

Species / Strain
It has long been suggested that cancer is species-specific (see Chapter 17 for information on which studies you can trust). All the data points in that direction; there is very little correlation to human effects from animal studies. Toxicology studies are difficult under such circumstances. But to be sure, err on the side of caution and avoid potential cancer-causing or toxic substances.

Genetic / Immune Status
Studies often use immune-impaired animals so that they'll be guaranteed of getting sick. Animal science is not quite an exact science. If you are immune impaired or genetically predisposed, you may be more susceptible to toxic substances.

Nutritional Status
Is your store of antioxidants sufficient to prevent the onslaughts of toxins? Do you get the correct amounts of the energy-yielding nutrients (fat, protein and carbohydrate), vitamins and minerals?

Stress
Stress is a factor in any disease. It may even be the precipitating event leading to toxicity or cancer. More on stress later.

Age/Sex/Weight
Young or very old animals are more susceptible to the ravages of toxins. Male animals have more immune problems. While excess weight causes a host of difficulties including fat storage of toxins, underweight animals can also be very susceptible to toxins.

Disease

The presence of disease in someone exposed to a toxin can seriously compromise their ability to deal with the toxin. The presence of multiple toxins, such as are found in cigarette smoke, makes detoxification of any single toxin that more difficult.

Environmental Factors That Affect Toxicity
Temperature
Humidity
Barometric Pressure
Ambient air
Light
Stress
Noise
Social Factors

Human Risk Factors

To assess the risk of a certain chemical or environmental factor causing harm, there are three major things to consider: the chemical or factor itself; the profile of the user of the substance; and the types of tests that are necessary.

Chemical Factors To Consider
Name
Structure
Formulas
Impurities
Physical / Chemical Properties
Manufacturing Conditions
Storage
Stability

Questions commonly asked by toxicologists to develop an <u>intake profile</u> include the following.

- How much of the substance is ingested, on average, at one time?
- How often is the substance ingested?
- Does the substance degrade?
- Are there degradation products?
- Who regularly ingests it?
- What are the advantages to the consumer?
- How carcinogenic (cancer causing) is it?
- What is the acute, chronic, genetic or reproductive toxicology of the substance (i.e., what are the observed effects)?

Food Interactions That Create Toxic Compounds

Combined Foods or Sources	Toxic Compound
Utensils / Plates	Heavy Metals
Colored Packaging	Heavy Metals
Protein & Sugar	Benzo(a)pyrene
Polyunsaturated Fatty Acids & Oxygen	Lipid Hydroperoxides
Bleach (in fish)	Chlorinated Lipids
Any food & excessive heat	Polycyclic Aromatics
Protein & Sugar	Premelanoidins

Food - Nutrient Interactions

Certain foods prevent the absorption of nutrients. The source of the interfering substance should be eaten separately from the compound with which it interferes. For example, whole grains contain phytates and bran, which can interfere with absorption of minerals.

Examples of Food - Nutrient Interactions		
Decreased Availability of	By	Source
Minerals	Phytates/Bran	Whole grains
Calcium	Protein	Meat, legumes
	Oxalates	Spinach, greens
Iodine	Goitrogens	Cruciferous vegetables
Iron	Polyphenols	Tea, red wine
Vitamins	Fiber	Plants
Biotin	Avidin	Raw egg
Thiamine	Thiaminases	Berries, shellfish
Protein	Ovomucoid	Eggs
	Protease Inhibitors	Legumes
Carbohydrate	Amylase Inhibitors	Legumes
Cholesterol	Saponins	Soy, alfalfa

Adapted from Rutgers University Food Science briefing

Cancer Causing Compounds in Foods

It is estimated that dietary factors account for more cancer deaths per year than any other single factor. This estimation includes tobacco (which is a close second!), infections, sexual behavior, occupation, alcohol, pollution, medicines and industrial products (Doll and Peto, 1981).

Cancer is largely attributable to the way we live, eat and drink. There are genetic factors to cancer as well, but you are powerless against your genes. Unlike hereditary factors, you can change your diet or your lifestyle.

Cancer is not always the result of one exposure or one food, but it can be. Meselthelioma (a special type of lung cancer) is one of the very few cancers that can be directly linked to a carcinogen, asbestos. Liver cancer can be the result of one poorly prepared fish or sushi dinner, because hepatitis acquired from this dinner can predispose the recipient to such an insult. Sex with someone infected with HPV or Human Papilloma Virus or Condylomata (genital warts) can directly result (for a woman) in death from cervical cancer sometime later. Other links are not as direct and hard, but compelling just the same. We know that almost all lung cancer and many tangential cancer cases (like bladder and esophageal) are the result of cigarette smoking or tobacco chewing. It is these links that we must break in order to prevent cancer.

Viruses help transfer information to cells and in so doing may be involved in many more cancer cases than originally suspected. We know about the common cold, the flu, and herpes viruses. But what do we know about viruses in our food? Very little. Oh, except for that virus (actually a small piece of renegade protein called a prion) that causes Mad Cow Disease! More on that later.

Is there transmission of chicken, beef or pork viruses or diseases **to our cells** from our food? There has been no clear demonstration except for Mad Cow Disease. And now Mad Cow Disease is not considered to be a virus. There is other evidence, however, that association with animals that are virally infected gives viruses the opportunity to infect our cells.

Don't blame the animals. And this is no reason to ditch the family pet. We do it to ourselves by not cleaning our hands and dishes properly. We do it to the animals we eat by keeping them in horrid, filthy squalor and squeezing them so close together that if one gets sick, they all do. This is the reason for the need for so much antibiotic in our meat supply. But the antibiotics work only for bacterial infections, not viral ones. And viruses cannot be heat killed under household circumstances all the time. In a study of cats with Feline Leukemia Virus, 69% of their owners tested positive for the antibody to this virus. And while this does not currently cause disease in humans, it is worth thinking about as far as virus ingression into our food and lives.

Meat inspectors have, for years, gone into packing plants and looked down the rows and said, "Looks good to me" as the final certification for the beef that you are about to eat! They can't **SEE** viruses, bacteria, prions or any other infective agents on the meat **WITHOUT A MICROSCOPE!!!** So we just go on our merry way with our steak tartare and rare prime rib assuming we're safe. Guess again. There is a shortage of meat inspectors in the U.S. and they <u>never will be able to look at even half</u> of the carcasses that pass by them and get their stamp of approval!

In fact, in one very recent five-year period, meat inspectors saw 644,076 beef carcasses with cancer, condemned 193,446 of them and sent 450,360 to be consumed! All they did was cut off the cancer they could see!!! We all know that cancer can metastasize and it could be present anywhere in the cow. We also know that cooking doesn't always kill viruses that cause cancer or unusual cell changes. Thirty different sarcoma viruses are present in chickens at commercial poultry houses. Carcinomas were found in 8% of flounder from Boston harbor, 50% of bullheads in certain areas of Pennsylvania, and in 80% of all fish in one polluted river in Wisconsin. (P. Lachance, 1989) Remember, now it is several years and many thousands of gallons of pollution later.

Food can help cause cancer by itself, or by working with other substances in a cumulative way in your body. A good example is FAT. There are many different theories about fat and cancer. I'll cut to the chase here. Excess saturated fat like butter, beef or pork fat, milk or cream is associated with fatty tissue cancers like breast, lymph and prostate cancer. Excess polyunsaturated fats like certain oils and margarine are associated with several other types of cancer. If we were talking about heart disease, the relationship would be different. Excess monounsaturated fats are not good for you either. The answer is to lower your lipid intake to less than 30 grams per day (shoot for 20 and miss) and to use oils high in monounsaturated fatty acids.

Fat in excess in your tissues offers more of a working area for oxidants to use as a place to deposit themselves. This "deposition" is actually more of the chemical reaction known as OXIDATION. It is not a good thing for your cells and can happen several ways and with several compounds. Fat provides a substrate for oxidants like smoke (cigarette, wood, industrial), barbecued meat compounds and other dangerous substances.

Thanksgiving Dinner Has Potentially Cancer-Causing Chemicals

Food	Compound
Cherry Tomato	Hydrogen peroxide, Quercetin glycoside, Nitrate
Tomato	Tomatine
Carrot	Myristicin, Isoflavones, Nitrate
Celery	Psoralens, Nitrate
Radishes	Nitrate
Mushroom Soup	Hydrazine
Stuffing	Hydrazine, Ethyl carbamate, Disulfides
Cranberry	Eugenol
Radishes	Glucosinolate
Broccoli	Glucosinolate, Goitrin, Allylisothionate, Nitrate
Potato	Isoflavones, Arsenic, Chaconine, Solanine
Apple Pie	Isoflavones, Quercetin glycoside, Acetaldehyde
Turkey	Heterocyclic amines, Malonaldehyde
Sweet Potato	Cyanogenic glycoside
Lima Beans	Cyanogenic glycoside
Fish	Arsenic
Pumpkin Pie	Myristicin, Eugenol, Safrole
Cheese	Tyramine
Herring	Tyramine
Rolls	Ethyl carbamate, Diacetyl
Coffee	Hydrogen peroxide, Caffeine, Tannins
Tea	Quercetin glycoside, Caffeine, Tannins
Red Wine	Ethyl carbamate, Tannins, Tyramine

Toxic Foods
To Wage War

Eat a variety of foods. This limits the amount of toxic compound you can get from any one food.

Eat only fresh foods. You will notice that many of the compounds found in the "Thanksgiving chart" are similar to the ones in the antioxidants chapter that follows. If you get them before they are oxidized they are good for you; if you get them after they are not.

Do not overcook foods. Many of the toxic compounds are created by excessive heat in combination with what might have been antioxidant compounds.

You may also want to check out Dr. Sherry Rodgers' publications like "Are Chemicals Making Me Sick?" and her "Total Health In Today's World" newsletter. For more information, call (800) 301-8970.

COUNTER
OFFENSIVES

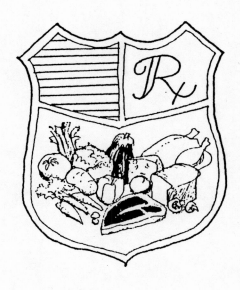

Chapter 15
ANTIOXIDANTS/
NUTRACEUTICALS

ANTIOXIDANTS

What is an "Antioxidant"? A compound that fights against an "Oxidant", or fights against "Oxidation". Oxidation, as we saw in the Lipids chapter, is the altering of the function or nature of a chemical substance. Most often it is the result of addition of positively charged compounds (ions) where they do not belong. It can also be a change created by heat, light, or other physical or chemical elements. If we eat them, these oxidized chemical compounds can then enter our cells and wreak havoc.

We have antioxidants in our foods to prevent spoilage. We eat antioxidant vitamins to prevent "spoilage" or cancer or disease in our bodies. Is there a relationship? You bet there is! Food antioxidants like BHA and BHT (Butylated hydroxy anisole and Butylated hydroxy toluene) which protect our food from spoiling CAUSE CANCER!!!

"What? I thought they were antioxidants!!!" They are; in your food!! But not in your body after they've worked in your food!! No one has caught on to this fact. The FDA is still so much in the dark that they are proposing to add BHA and BHT to vitamins in the near future. Don't panic yet. There's more to the story.

"Why do antioxidants BHA and BHT cause Cancer?"

SECRET # 1 About Antioxidants

THEY ARE PRO-OXIDANTS IF OXIDIZED!!!

The key to preventing or causing cancer with these compounds is **the state of oxidation the compounds are in.** In other words, how much of their antioxidant capacity is used up and turned into pro-oxidant activity before you eat them? You need to know this. It is vitally important to your health.

Oxidation Questions

Why can Vitamin C give you cancer if taken with Iron?

Why is beta-carotene an antioxidant, but Vitamin A is a potential pro-oxidant?

Why did even Beta-carotene actually accelerate lung cancer in a recent long-term Finnish study?

Why should you throw out old vitamins and old medications?

Why can eating old crackers give you cancer?

Why do people who smoke menthol cigarettes have higher incidences of serious and aggressive cancers than regular smokers?

THE ANSWER? OXIDATION

You need to make sure that the foods and chemicals you eat are in a form as close to the original food they were derived from to prevent as much unnatural oxidation as possible. This, of course, means that we'll have to be a bit more diligent about food storage because fewer preservatives means quicker degradation of foods.

We'll have to eat them quicker, but in return we'll live longer, healthier lives.

Vitamin C and Iron

Iron is known as a strong pro-oxidant. Too much iron in your system can cause excess microbial growth, cancer, and even precipitate symptoms from a rare genetic disorder known as Hemochromatosis in which your organs are successively destroyed. But take your iron with Vitamin C and you have even more trouble. Vitamin C binds iron fairly easily, which is why we've been told for years to take iron supplements with orange juice for better absorption. And it does give you better absorption. It also gives you a Vitamin C molecule chemically bound to iron, ready to integrate itself into the cytoplasm of your cells, in an OXIDIZED form!!! And we know what that means! Vitamin C and iron together are a very powerful pro-oxidant!

Beta-Carotene Versus Vitamin A

Structurally, Vitamin A and beta-carotene look very much alike; Vitamin A is almost exactly half of the Beta-carotene molecule. Both compounds have the same ring structure and an isoprenoid tail. What, then, is the difference? My conjecture, and that's all it is at this point, is that Vitamin A is heavily oxidized or "used up" by the time you ingest it in vitamin or even food form.

Why? Well, Vitamin A is an animal compound; never found in plants. It is always isolated from animal storage organs, mainly the liver. The liver, as we know, is the main detoxifying organ of the body. If you're an excessive drinker or pill taker, hopefully you'll never find out the limits of your liver to detoxify all of the junk you give it. If you're exposed to environmental insults such as toxic organic compounds or viruses, your liver is also at the ready to do what it can to remove them. Over the years, or with repeated insults, your liver may not be able to keep up, in which case toxins may build up. Livers can be full of junk that cannot be detoxified.

When we eat some animal's liver, we are potentially exposing ourselves to any or all of the toxins and viruses it has come in contact with during its lifetime. [In the chapter on Food Safety there is a discussion of how animals are raised and what they eat.] It could be a very dangerous thing to eat liver. Kiss the pate good-bye.

Right about now you're feeling pretty good for hating liver long before I mentioned this, but wait. Vitamin A is isolated from all kinds of livers, including fish liver. We usually don't force fish to eat awful toxins like we do our livestock. They can eat what they like. They're swimming free in the ocean before we kill them for dinner.

But is it a healthy environment to live in? Answer me this (non-septic tank owners); do you know where the flushes of your toilet go? Yes, you and all of the millions of people who flush and forget everyday. The ultimate destination is THE OCEAN!!! Would you eat a fish that fell in your toilet? No. But you'll gladly have your Vitamin A taken from the liver of a fish who has been swimming around in feces, garbage, hepatitis viruses, etc. His liver is taking in all of this and desperately trying to detoxify it. And, no, the fishing boats don't all go out far enough in the ocean to catch fresh, clean fish. There is no "out far enough in the ocean" anymore. We're running out of ocean water to pollute. Back to my theory.

When Vitamin A is taken from fish liver, it can not be completely isolated from the oxidants that are present in that liver. Some divalent cations (like iron and other minerals) or compounds that have attached themselves to the Vitamin A molecule will likely end up in your Vitamin A pill. This does not mean that all manufacturers of Vitamin A are irresponsible; they just don't have this information and it would be very expensive to isolate absolutely pure Vitamin A anyway.

O.K. Perhaps Vitamin A can be toxic or cancer-causing, but Beta-carotene? Beta-carotene has not been inside a liver and is a plant compound. How could IT be toxic or accelerate cancer as in the Finnish study? Once again, OXIDATION is the probable answer. Whenever you take a food and subdivide it into its components, oxidation can result. Exposure to heat, light, or certain positively charged minerals can result in an antioxidant becoming a pro-oxidant. Eat a fresh carrot and you're O.K.; take a Beta-carotene pill and who knows? There are also other lipid-soluble compounds that might take a ride with Beta-carotene when it's isolated. Pesticides. Residue from certain pesticides might be present in that Beta-carotene pill and cause you problems later on. And you don't know where that carrot was grown. ("We have the largest three-pronged carrots in the world right here at Nuclear Farms!")

Old Vitamins
Pharmaceutical companies do their best to protect your vitamins from oxidation once you receive them by using light-excluding packaging, dessicants and cotton. This prevents some oxidation while you have the vitamins in your own care. But no amount of protection can prevent the ravages of time. Old vitamins and old medications have not just "lost potency" - they've become oxidized.

Old Crackers
"You must be joking." Actually I'm not. Old cookies, crackers, and biscuits can expose you to several toxic compounds that are a result of, again, OXIDATION.

"Wait, there's nothing to oxidize; crackers are just flour and salt!" And LIPIDS!! A major player in the oxidized cookie realm is a group of compounds known as **Epoxides**. These are formed as a result of lipid oxidation and are powerful pro-oxidants that can affect your cells permanently.

Throw out the old crackers, cookies, and old pet biscuits! Pet cancer and illnesses result from very much the same insults as we have. Any way you look at it, the risk isn't worth it.

Menthol Cigarettes
Anecdotal information derived from studies of smokers suggests that smokers of menthol cigarettes get much more aggressive cancers than those who smoke regular cigarettes. Wait, menthol is also an antioxidant! Shouldn't it be more protective? No. Remember that antioxidants that are oxidized, for example by the many hazardous compounds in cigarette smoke, are almost a vector for oxidants to your cells! It is the state of oxidation that counts here. If it's oxidized, don't eat, drink or smoke it!

In fact, listen to any information on the TV or radio about something that causes cancer and ask yourself how close that "something" is to its natural state; you'll be able to see what I mean by Antioxidant Secret #1!

SECRET # 2 About Antioxidants

MOST IMPORTANT IS THE ISOPRENOID UNIT

A majority of the compounds that are of nutraceutical/antioxidant value have isoprenoid units. The **isoprenoid unit** is a small chemical compound that gives great antioxidant benefits. Beta-carotene has a long isoprenoid unit between its two ring structures. Any monoterpenoid compound is actually two isoprenoid units hooked together. Mint, rosemary and pine compounds that are mono-, di-, and tri-terpenoid compounds are composed of several isoprenoid units. Many other compounds include isoprenoids as well.

The isoprenoid unit has amazing quenching power when it comes to pro-oxidants. Oxidants can be held and passed down a long isoprenoid tail, or picked up by the double bond in just one single unit. The isoprenoid unit has great potential to de-oxidize our cells, but as I said before, not in isolation. All important compounds should be acquired from food.

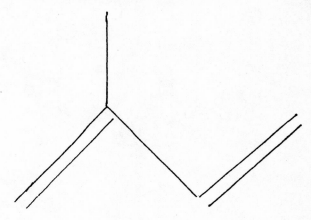

The Isoprenoid Unit

SECRET # 3 About Antioxidants

Below is a diagram of exactly where in the typical cell in your body, these compounds can go. The difference in location has a lot to do with their solubility in fatty or lipid substances and their electrical charge. We can see that Beta-carotene crosses the entire lipid membrane, because it is very fat-soluble, while Vitamin C is usually found inside the cell (in the cytoplasm) due to its water solubility.

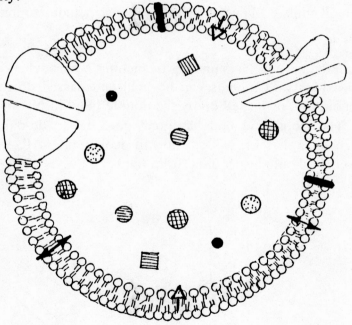

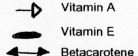

Vitamin A

Vitamin E

Betacarotene

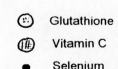

Glutathione

Vitamin C

Selenium

Components of DNA Damage and Cancer

DNA Damage

DNA, as explained in the Cell section, is the "Brain" of your cells. It determines exactly what goes on and what doesn't. If you damage this DNA in one cell, it can repeat over and over again and turn into a cancer cell, making copies of itself faster than the normal cells that surround it. This is tumor initiation.

DNA is a ladder-shaped chemical with many atoms glued together in a very organized fashion. Assume this DNA is a wooden ladder for this analogy. This ladder can have a rung break as if someone too heavy for the ladder had stepped on it, a side snap from some impact (**strand break**), an old rung repaired with an odd kind of wood (**base modification**), one step fall onto another and stay (**pyrimidene dimers**), or extra wood lengths inserted (**intercalation**). All these types of damage can and do occur both due to outside forces such as mutagens and spontaneously without provocation. Most of the time your DNA calls on the local handyman to repair it. The removal of damaged steps or of half of a damaged step begins with **nucleotide excision** by handyman enzymes called **endo or exonucleases**.

Cancer is a multistep process. It depends on many factors including age, exercise, exposure and genetic predisposition to repair. If you're like George Burns, the comedian who lived to 100 and did all the wrong things (note, though, that he exercised every day of his life!), then you probably have a genetic repair system that works like a charm. Unfortunately the only way to test it is to live hard and mess yourself up and see if you can recover. Not a prescription for happiness and good health for most of us!

DNA: The Double Helix

This is a piece of DNA. It is very much like the ladder described in the text, but more like a rope ladder. You will notice the Bases as steps in the ladder (A,T,G,C). These are the basic building blocks. If these are disrupted in any way, mutation and disease can result. Below we show three types of damage your DNA can suffer.

First we have Ultraviolet Radiation which has created a Thymine dimer (two of the base "T"s stuck together). This can happen anytime you are exposed to the sun or fluorescent light. Next we show what can happen if you eat peanut butter or corn contaminated with Aflatoxin. Aflatoxin imitates the base Guanine (G) and inserts itself in your DNA. Cancer is not an unusual result. Lastly we have a typical chemical found in barbequed food, Benzo-a-pyrene. This can insert between the bases and create havoc when cells go to divide and make new cells.

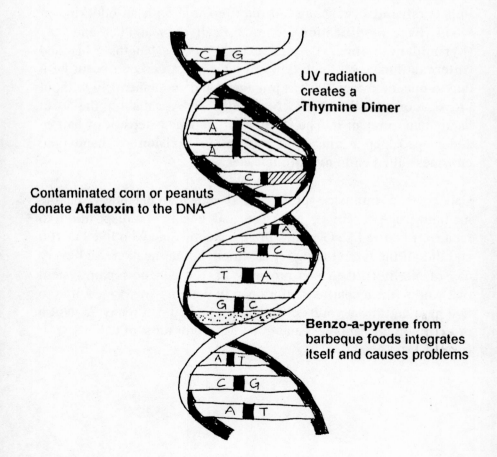

UV radiation creates a **Thymine Dimer**

Contaminated corn or peanuts donate **Aflatoxin** to the DNA

Benzo-a-pyrene from barbeque foods integrates itself and causes problems

In "Antimutagens As Chemopreventive Agents In The Diet" (Ferguson, 1994) in Mutation Research, it is suggested that there will be several future functions of antioxidants/antimutagens in our diets. The first is in direct prevention of cancer and genetic disease. This would include interference in DNA repair, mutagen metabolism, and as a mutagen scavenger. All of these functions might have positive outcomes if we paired, as suggested in this article, the mutagens with their antimutagen.

Certain antioxidant compounds have been labeled **Desmutagens** and **Bio-Antimutagens**. **Desmutagens** (Kada, 1995) prevent either the formation of the mutagen or the metabolic interaction with your DNA with inactivation of the important components of the mutagen. **Bio-Antimutagens** block the damaged DNA from remaining mutant and causing cancer or genetic difficulties.

There is great potential for disaster in this, however. Antioxidants are also pro-oxidants if given the right set of circumstances. Dr. Victor Herbert (Mt. Sinai School of Medicine, in a 1995 speech) was one of the first people to sound the alarm. At the time he suggested that beta-carotene promoted cervical cancer in women, it wasn't known exactly why. My theory goes one step further and states that any antioxidant (phytochemical, nutraceutical, etc.) can be changed back and forth from Good (if you will) to Bad with the removal or application of oxidants. This includes during vitamin manufacturing, vitamin storage, and even in the green plant source.

These phytochemical antioxidants serve to protect green plants from the ravages of pro-oxidants like the UV rays of sunlight, which plants desperately need, and from pollutants. Part of my idea that **you need to know the state of oxidation of your antioxidant** is that it might change even before being put into pill form, for example, in a plant under stress. If the source of your beta-carotene is carrots from a farm at the edges of an industrial city with large amounts of sulfur or nitrogen dioxides, particulates, or other air pollutants, it might end up being "used up" or oxidized. It is worth knowing where your produce comes from. But if the source of the compound or produce is fine, the isolation and manufacturing of a product containing this compound might not be fine.

Packaging and Shipping
Oxidants can be added during isolation, packaging, shipping and storage. Shipping? Yes, there are stories of shipments of chocolate chip cookies that were rejected because they had absorbed too much volatile compounds from the spilled oil that their palette was placed on through their thin packaging. This is a case where the manufacturer was being conscientious. There are times, though, that the manufacturer might not be able to catch a shipment that has been oxidized or exposed to toxics. That happens during one of the worst, most ignorant abuses of shipping that occurs today. The backhaul.

If you're a trucker, then you know what I'm talking about. Let me explain it for the rest of us non-truckers. When you drive a shipment of food, it goes from, let's say, California to New York; you get paid for your California to New York trip. You get nothing for the trip back home. That's called the backhaul. Let me say for the record right now, that most truck drivers are very conscientious and would never do what I'm about to tell you, but it does happen more often than we'd like to believe.

Let's say someone's trucking a product from the West coast to the East. That person would like not to lose the gas and time costs on the way back, but there is often nothing to haul back. If the trucker owns his/her truck, he/she can pick up anything else from almost any sort of manufacturer! There are few controls set up to monitor this in spite of the fact that it has been going on for many years.

The truck can be filled with food again the next day. Another problem is that a trucker who doesn't understand that you can't clean out all of the toxic compounds with one cursory rinse is then putting them into all subsequent loads of food. All that is needed is proper pay to cover the backhaul, monitoring and more education about the dangers and the criminal nature of hauling toxins in food containers.

There is also the great potential (it happens every day) that your food might have absorbed toxic or cancer-causing compounds from the packaging. Much of our packing is made with poly-vinyl compounds which attach themselves to any foods with soluble components or fat. Foods like baked goods can also be in contact with colored packaging which has toxic metals that will migrate into the food.

Milk, for example, is becoming a concern. Either you can drink it out of the plastic containers that donate their volatile compounds to the fat portion of the milk (I can always taste it) or you can drink it from a container made with paraffin (another toxic compound). I go with paraffin because I am not organoleptically aware of the funny taste like plastic-containered milk has. The best way to get milk is from inert glass or steel containers. Ah, maybe we need to bring the milkman back!

But all packaging has potential to donate harmful synthetic compounds to your food.

Tumor Promotion

Tumor promotion does not take place in isolation. It is an event that has several stages prior to metastasis. Below are four phases prior to tumor promotion and the nutraceutical compounds that prevents the phase from progressing to tumor promotion. These phases follow the development of breast cancer. (Pierson, 1992 / Lachance 1994).

1.   Oxidative Damage

We encounter oxidants on a daily basis. Oxidation is the reason metal rusts and our hair turns gray. Many times our defenses can prevent injury to our cells, but certain nutraceutical compounds can help. Damage resulting from several oxidative compounds can be prevented from promoting tumor growth with carotenoids, phenolics, terpenes, tocopherols, and flavonoids.

2.   Initiation

The initiation site is the point where a carcinogen is introduced and could start a tumor. It has been found that cells rich in certain compounds can prevent tumor formation. Let's say you're worried about the benzo(a)pyrene found in barbecued meat. It doesn't mean that you can eat a barbecued burger (and at the same time) drink a glass of orange juice and it'll be OK... Although a researcher recently found that a marinade containing orange juice, olive oil, garlic, and cider vinegar prevented formation of the carcinogenic compounds in barbecued meat...It means that you need a diet rich in foods that contain nutraceutical compounds all the time, because you never know when the assaults will come.

Coumarins, flavonoids, and tri-terpenoids are the main compounds that will prevent an assault by a known carcinogen from becoming an initiation site. **Vitamins C and E** are also known to help in this regard. Remember, though, that Vitamin E comes in several forms and while we have always thought that **alpha tocopherol** was the most active, that concept is now being challenged because it appears that **gamma tocopherol** has active properties as well. A group of mixed tocopherols might serve best. Once a tumor has been initiated, **sulfides (garlic, onion compounds)** and **isoflavones** are known to inhibit its growth.

3.   Prostaglandin (PGS)

Prostaglandin synthesis is necessary for several body functions, but also helps enhance tumor growth. This may be the reason that aspirin helps lower the risk of colon cancer, because aspirin interferes with prostaglandin formation. The nutraceutical compounds that prevent prostaglandin interference in tumor promotion are **phenolics, salicylates (aspirin, birch bark tea), flavonoids, polyacetylenes, and sulfides.**

4.   Steroid Hormones

Ingested steroids are heavily associated with cancers and disease. But we couldn't exist without our ever-present *natural* steroids. They are important to our health and development Unfortunately, though, they also can enhance and promote tumor development. The nutraceutical compounds which prevent steroid promotion of tumor growth are **fibers, phytosterols, terpenes, sulfides, phenolics, lignans, isoflavones, tri-terpenoids, cruciferous indoles (like Indole-3-Carbinol from broccoli).**

Foods Which Prevent Cancer - Nutraceuticals

Nutraceuticals, Pharmafoods, Antioxidants, Phytochemicals, Designer or Engineered Foods are all names for a remarkable group of compounds or foods made with these compounds. They all are foods or compounds which capitalize on the properties of plants that have been found to enhance our lives and prevent disease and cancer. Some of these foods have long histories of medicinal use as folk remedies. Nutritional science is just beginning to catch up and recognize many of these as important components of a disease-free diet.

The "properties" of these substances that we take advantage of are actually plant chemical substances which integrate into our tissues, providing us with healthy cells and preventing OXIDATION. It is oxidation which starts us on the path to cancerous tumors. It starts with very small changes in your cells and the end result can be cells which grow uncontrollably and cannot be stopped. That is what is known as cancer.

We now know many foods or chemicals in foods that really can make a difference. We do not have to get cancer!

Prevent	By Eating Foods With
Oxidation	Carotenoids, phenolics, terpenes, tocopherols, flavonoids
Tumor initiation	Coumarins, flavonoids, tocopherols, triterpenoids
Spreading of tumor	Sulfides, isoflavones,polyacetylenes, phenolics, salicylates
Hormonal tumor growth	Fiber,lignans, indoles, phytosterols, terpenes, sulfides, phenolics,isoflavones

Major Nutraceuticals and the Foods Which Contain Them

Sulfides	Garlic, cruciferous vegetables
Phytates	Soybeans, grains
Flavonoids	All tea, almost all vegetables
Glucarates	Green tea, grains, citrus fruits, cruciferous, solanaceous
Carotenoids	Soybeans, cucurbitaceous, citrus Grains, cruciferous, umbelliferous Solanaceous
Coumarins	All vegetables but garlic
Mono-terpenes	Mint, garlic, rosemary, citrus Cucurbitaceous, cruciferous Umbelliferous, solanaceous
Tri-terpenes	All from mono group plus garlic Soy, grains, and licorice
Lignans	Soybeans, flax seed
Phenolic compounds	All plants
Indoles	Cruciferous
Isothiocyanates	Cruciferous
Phthalides	Umbelliferous
Polyacetylenes	Umbelliferous

Key to Vegetable Groups:

Solanaceous	Potatoes, tomatoes, peppers
Cruciferous	Broccoli, cabbage, cauliflower
Cucurbitaceus	Cucumbers, etc
Umbelliferous	Celeriac root, parsnip, etc.

Examples of Nutraceutical Compounds

SOY + PHYTOESTROGENS
Dr. Steven Barnes of University of Alabama wrote about the protective effects of dietary soy compounds on breast cancer in "Soy component Genistein may protect against breast cancer" (Food Chem. News, 1994, pp. 62). Genestein is a phytoestrogen, one of several found in soy products. Phytoestrogens are compounds analogous to mammalian estrogen, which target cells that respond to estrogen. Other plants like rye seed also contain phytoestrogens.

In Barnes' study, the rate of breast cancer in Asian women recently arriving in this country increased the longer they stayed and ate a western diet. The protective nature of the soy products that they had eaten all their lives in Asia continued to provide protection for a time. Non-Asian women consuming soy products with high Genistein saw a beneficial effect when compared with Western women with Western diets. Phytoestrogen effects were the main reason.

Tofu has much more Genistein than soy sauce, but other products like soy protein isolate, soy molasses, defatted soy, and soy flour showed beneficial effects as well. Soy products also contain Diadzein, another phytoestrogen. Soy butter may be better for you than peanut butter, if you are concerned about getting enough phytoestrogens. Dr. Barnes also found protective effects (a two- to six-fold decrease) against prostate cancer and leukemia. Soy consumption could be more important than a low fat diet as a single factor in breast cancer prevention. It is, however, still very important to follow a low fat diet.

FLAX

Lignans are protective compounds that can be created in mammals after ingestion of plant analogs. Flax is a rich source of these lignan compounds. Mammalian lignans are called Enterodiol and Enterolactone. Lignans and flax can slow the progression of kidney disease, control prostaglandin and inflammatory events, and influence hormonally independent cancer.

Flax also contains two compounds that are very much in the news now, Omega-3 and Omega-6 essential oils. While they can be obtained from fish, flax has them in a better proportion. It is better to have more Omega-3 than Omega-6. "Designer eggs" are currently being developed that will have more Omega-3 in them. The chickens are being given flax seed in their feed.

GARLIC

Garlic (*Allium sativum*) has been recognized as a healthful root since at least 3000 B.C. It has been used by all civilizations that had access to it including the Egyptians, Babylonians, Greeks, Romans, Vikings, Indians, Chinese and all knowledgeable Western and European civilizations. Garlic undisputedly offers health advantages. These properties are is being considered by researchers around the world.

The compounds in garlic that are most active are alliin, allicin, ajoene, diallyl sulfide, and methyl allyl trisulfide. Of the many reported beneficial effects, those which have scientific backing include:

- Reduced serum lipids
- Reduced atherosclerotic lesions
- Anticoagulant (Blood thinning) properties
- Antibacterial properties

(1 milligram of garlic has 1% penicillin activity)
- Antiviral properties
- Inhibits platelet aggregation in the test tube
- Antitumor properties
  (stomach, skin, prostate, breast, colon and esophagus)
- Immunomodulatory properties
- Antineoplastic properties (inhibits initial tumor site)

The active compounds in garlic can be obtained in several ways. **Garlic oil** can be manufactured by steam distillation (producing diallyl disulfide). **Garlic powder** is obtained by ethanol-water extraction or by crushing (Allicin). An **aged extract (5% active compounds)** is also produced by cold ethanol extraction (Alliin).

Before you put yourself on an all-garlic diet, be warned that excessively high intake can precipitate anemia, weight loss, dermatitis, and asthma. High garlic intake can also cause bleeding in patients on anticoagulants such as coumarins or salicylates, or can cause problems in those that need blood glucose regulation.

TEA / BLACK

Black tea, first exchanged for decaffeinated and later herbal teas, may not be so bad for us after all. The presence of caffeine indicates that the other phenolic compounds are mostly intact, and when considering antioxidant effects, this is most important. Black tea from *Camellia* leaves contains catechins which are enzymatically oxidized to become Theaflavins and Thearubigens (two good antioxidant compounds) in the production process. In a recent study in Denmark, it was found that those who drank a few cups of black tea or ate apples each day often were protected against heart trouble and cancer. Could it be that "an apple (or cup of tea) a day" really does keep the doctor away? According to all we currently know, yes! But make it an organic, well-washed apple for the best effect.

Black tea prevents cavities! Especially if you don't sweeten it too much or add too much milk. The theaflavins and thearubigens in the tea, along with other phenolics and caffeine, also have antimicrobial effects in your mouth and inhibit the formation of cavities.

Some major Theaflavins in black tea include:
    TF1
    TF Monogallate A (TF2A)
    TF Monogallate B (TF2B)
    TF Digallate (TF3)

Oolong tea is intermediate between black and green tea and retains many catechins due to partial oxidation.

Earl Grey Tea is a regular black tea with an added antioxidant, originally added not as an antioxidant but as a flavoring. The antioxidant is bergamot oil from the leaves of wild bergamot or purple beebalm (*Monarda fistulosa*). Bergamot is related to other antioxidants like mint and rosemary oil. Its protective effects are assumed to be similar to those compounds; more preventative of oxidation than curative after the fact.

TEA / GREEN
Everyone's heard about Green Tea and its cancer preventing abilities. What exactly does it do? Manufactured from the fresh leaves of the same plant that black tea comes from, *Camellia sinensis*, green tea undergoes little processing and therefore has its polyphenols (catechins) preserved from oxidation.

There are four major Green Tea Catechins:
Epicatechin	EC
Epigallocatechin	EGC
Epicatechin Gallate	ECG
Epigallocatechin Gallate	EGCG

These catechins are effective against the carcinogens to which we are exposed as a result of air pollution, cigarette smoke, and barbecued meat. They can serve as a preventative measure prior to exposure to such carcinogens.

Green tea affects tumor initiation. Its catechins block the formation of carcinogens in the body, inhibit metabolic activation of carcinogens, stimulate DNA repair, and actually bind to DNA preferentially over the carcinogens mentioned. This binding forms a physical block to the integration of cancer-causing compounds in your cells.

Green tea appears to affect tumor promotion by inhibiting a compound called TPA. TPA produces H_2O_2 (Hydrogen peroxide), active oxygen species, and oxidized DNA bases (like Thymine glycol and 8 Hydroxydeoxyguanine). TPA also creates skin hyperplasia (growths). In short, green tea can stop promotion of tumors.

TEA / HERBAL
Herbal teas can be mixtures of pure substances, flavoring and black tea. However, a true herbal blend will not have added flavorants or black tea in the mix. For example, peppermint tea comes in many forms, but pure peppermint tea contains only leaves of *Mentha piperita*. These leaves contain several antioxidant compounds including thymol and menthol. A good, unfettered tea manufacturer is Celestial Seasonings™. They have herbal tea that

has no additives or flavorings, as well as regular tea with flavorings. Explore the possibilities.

BROCCOLI
Sulforaphane and Indole-3-carbinol are among the potentially anti-cancer, antioxidant, phytoestrogenic compounds in broccoli. Heated broccoli may release more of these compounds than raw broccoli. Other cruciferous vegetables like brussels sprouts, cabbage, broccoli sprouts and cauliflower have many of these compounds as well.

Forbidden Foods That Are Good For You

I hope you'll be as happy as I was to learn that nutraceuticals and antioxidants turn up in "forbidden" foods - the ones we love but have been told are "bad" for us. This is not a license to go overboard on any of these foods, but a little bit here and there may be more than just O.K. - it may be just what the doctor ordered.

LICORICE
The Licorice root, *Glycyrrhiza glabra,* has been used to flavor candy and foods for many years. Recently the antioxidant and therapeutic effects of licorice have been enumerated in scientific journals.

Licorice contains triterpenoid compounds which are large multiple isoprenoid units. These antioxidant compounds bind estrogen receptor sites and prevent possible precancerous interactions between estrogen and susceptible cells. The isoflavones found in licorice inhibit proteins produced by oncogenes *in vitro* (cancer genes in the laboratory). However, glycyrrhizin, while serving several good functions, may elevate blood pressure as well.

COFFEE

Caffeine is an antioxidant. Yes, it has the same phenolic potential to be antioxidant as all other related compounds. Once again, the trick is its oxidational status. Reheated cups of coffee, old tins of coffee grounds, and any long stay on the shelf can affect these properties adversely. Over time, coffee compounds become pro-oxidants or potent mutagens, like every other antioxidant mentioned. So sniff and drink FRESH cups of coffee and tea and enjoy the benefits of an antioxidant you never knew existed.

WINE

In "The effect of red and white wine on serum lipids, platelet aggregation, oxidation products, and antioxidants: A preliminary report" (Struck et al, 1994), it was suggested that there is an antithrombogenic (anticlotting) and antioxidant effect from both red and white wine. LDL cholesterol was lowered and antioxidant potential appeared to be greater for white wine in this study.

More recent studies have shown Resveratrol in red wine (and grape juice/raisins) to have great potential cholesterol lowering properties. This compound appears to be produced by grapes as a mechanism to fight disease. According to Barbara Frank, of Vinifera Wine Cellars and Chateau Frank, the Chateau Frank Pinot Noir has the highest concentration of resveratrol of any red wine (46 micromolar, versus an average concentration of 0.1 to 12). Purple grape juice averages 0.2 to 4.0 micromolar resveratrol, but if you make it at home it can be as high as any red wine. Studies conducted by Professor L.L. Creasy at Cornell University confirm this.

I have long speculated that the heart disease prevention capabilities of wine are a result of the antimicrobial effect of alcohol in the blood more than the effect of other antioxidant compounds. If this is true, it might behoove those at risk for heavy bacterial infections to consume small amounts of alcohol as a preventative of infection. Dental patients with continuing decay problems might do well to consider this concept. After all, most mouthwash is alcohol-based, containing menthol and eucalyptol.

While it is generally accepted that people with periodontal disease are at much greater risk of heart disease and clotting problems, the reason is seldom discussed. It's the infection they have in their mouths that becomes disseminated system-wide. They don't necessarily have septicemia or heavy levels of the bacteria that often opens the door to dental decay (like *Streptococcus mutans*) in their blood or anything, they have just enough infection to start hidden damage to vessels. Bacteria and possibly viral ingression into the cells lining our blood vessels and our blood stream can create damage to vessels and leave an opening for clots to form. Wine may help offset this infection by killing bacteria and some viruses.

BRAZIL NUTS
Loaded with the antioxidant mineral selenium, brazil nuts are the best way to get this nutrient. Supplements are considered dangerous. Selenium has several beneficial effects; mood elevation, HDL raising, liver damage prevention and improved thinking (according to a recent study). It works in concert with Vitamin E and glutathione in your cells to prevent oxidation of cellular molecules. While there is a protective effect, it appears that selenium may also enhance certain cancers, while protecting against others.

MINTS AND MINT CANDY
Mints, especially Peppermint, have wonderful antioxidant abilities. Menthol and Thymol are two of the mint compounds that provide these benefits. Both are monoterpene compounds. Monoterpenes are also di-isoprenoid units (mentioned in the beginning of the

antioxidant section).   It is this isoprene connection that makes antioxidants so powerful.

Mints also have antimicrobial capabilities that may render them helpful during cold or flu season. I personally have tested the antimicrobial properties on myself during a close association with a large group of sick singers, whose breathing exudates I regularly inhaled. When you're with singers, you all share lung and mouth bacteria whether you want to or not. Sick myself for the first year I was with them, I later decided to always have a menthol throat lozenge in my mouth when I was near the singers. Perhaps it was the aeration of the antimicrobial menthol compound (you can always feel the sensation throughout your nose and lungs), my awakened awareness of disease transmission, or the placebo effect. But it always works for me. And the first men who insisted upon sanitary conditions in surgery, Ignaz Sammelweiss and Oliver Wendell Holmes, used a menthol cousin (carbolic acid) sprayed in the operating room and it worked!

CHOCOLATE
Chocolate is a food that many of us indulge in. We have been told to avoid such foods if our goal is long life and good health. And chocolate is fat-rich, so care needs to be taken that we not eat too very much of it. But, happily, there is another side to this story; one involving phenolics and phenylethylamine.

Phenolic compounds - Chocolate, it turns out, is rich in phenolic antioxidant compounds that, like red wine (which contains Resveratrol), help prevent heart and circulatory problems like atherosclerosis and the initiation of cancer. It is the cocoa that contains these compounds, so the benefit is derived from chocolates that contain the most cocoa and are often the most expensive. Chocolates that are inexpensive often have fillers like paraffin (potentially toxic and cancer-causing) which negate the benefits.

Tooth Decay Prevention - Chocolate may also prevent tooth decay. It is the compounds like caffeine and other phenolics that mutate bacteria like <u>*Streptococcus mutans*</u>, a known cavity-causer, and prevent them from setting up shop in your mouth. Once again, it is the cocoa-rich chocolates that are the ones that have the most benefit.

Immune-Enhancing Properties - While this is currently a stretch, there is some evidence to suggest that chemicals which alleviate stress and provide an individual with relaxation can enhance immune function. Such chemicals, akin to the endorphins and encephalins normally found in the brain, are found in chocolate. Phenylethylamine is one such compound. Known for several years to produce feelings of relaxation and pleasure, it has been touted as the "love" chemical by several popular magazines. While not inducive of such emotional feelings, it is nevertheless a compound which merits consideration as a relaxation-inducing substance.

It has also been suggested by several studies that those who use caffeine (from coffee, chocolate, tea, or other substances) are less likely to suffer the ravages of severe depression. Now this is only a suggestion at this point. If you abuse a drug like caffeine long enough, bad things will happen, like lack of ability to sleep, irritability, etc. So while you avoid serious depression, no one wants to be with someone cranky, so go easy.

Antioxidants/Nutraceuticals
To Wage War

1) Throw out old vitamins. If they are oxidized, they can give you cancer.

2) Avoid foods with preservatives that are antioxidants (BHA, BHT). These can also be carcinogenic.

3) Eat whole foods, not prepared foods, whenever possible.

4) Eat an apple every day (wash it well), or have a cup of tea for the phenolic compounds.

5) Eat a carrot every day for its fiber and beta-carotene.

6) If you want to take antioxidants, check for the vegetables and fruits in which they are found. Eat the vegetables and fruits instead of taking pills.

Chapter 16
HEALING STRATEGIES

"You can feed her all day with the Vitamin A and the bromo-fizz,
but the medicine never seems to end up where the trouble is..."
- from the musical Guys and Dolls

The Clipboard

A friend of mine recently told a cautionary tale about being diagnosed with sarcoma. He was quite taken by surprise with this pronouncement, as many people are, and waited for the other shoe to drop. "How did this happen?" he wondered. He waited for the doctor with the clipboard.

Having been transferred from another hospital to a famous New York cancer treatment center, he was expecting the doctor with the clipboard who asks, "So, tell me about your history...Exposed to any environmental carcinogens? Having any other crises in your life? What do you eat?..." But, alas, such an individual never showed up. In fact, he soon realized that such an individual does not exist. "But why not?", he asked. "I wanted to know how I got this! I wanted to have my personal information help prevent someone else from getting this!"

Your cancer treatment, using traditional medicine, will consist of being poisoned, burned, or surgically mutilated. In some respects, medicine has evolved little from the Middle Ages, with the exception of the addition of a few electronic gadgets. Most physicians are not well educated in the association between environmental or nutritional encounters and disease, and therefore do not wish to even discuss it with you. The imperious and uncaring phrases they use tell the story. "Just take off your clothes and lie down...Roll over...(Fetch)...You may lose your hair in a few days...You only have 6 months to live." They are afraid to discuss what they do not understand and will put you off if you try to ask how you came to have cancer.

My only answer to the clipboard dilemma is to have you interrupt the doctor while he/she is taking your "history" and make sure he/she includes all of the relevant information you think might relate to your cancer.

Aging

Why We Age

Aging is the result of several processes, including the two most often discussed lately, Oxidation and Glycosylation. Oxidation is the changing of compounds to make them more vulnerable to breakdown, as in the graying of hair, rusting of metal or the unrestrained growth of cancer. Oxidation is discussed in the previous chapter on Antioxidants. Glycosylation is the result of the end products of what food scientists call the Maillard (pronounced MY-ard) reaction.

 The Maillard reaction is the heat induced linking of an amino acid (often lysine) and a sugar. It is thought that this reaction occurs slowly over time in our 98.6°F bodies. The gooey brown stuff that tastes so wonderful when we brown onions is the same sort of sticky mess that can form inside our joints, organs and brain. The products of this glycosylation are referred to as AGE (Advanced Glycosylated End products). These globs of glycosylation are also often found in the brains of patients with Altzheimers disease, although scientists do not think they are the main cause of the brain's breakdown.

Maillard / Glycosylation Effects In Your Food

Flavor is enhanced. The Maillard reaction occurs whenever there is non-enzymatic or heat-induced browning in food. The browning of onions, butter, and meats occurs when we cook them. Some of the products are very tasty.

Color is produced. The production of the most overused coloring, caramel color, is derived almost exclusively from the Maillard reaction. Check the packages of everything you suspect of being colored and I'll bet you will find caramel coloring.

Texture is changed. A gooey, sticky substance results when combining an amino acid and sugar under heat. This substance can be used to add texture to certain foods such as gravy.

Toxic and cancerous compounds result. Carmel coloring is only one of the many products of the Maillard reaction which are toxic and cancer promoting. There are many others. When the amino acids phenylalanine or tryptophan react with glucose, they produce several of these compounds. They do not have to be under direct heat conditions such as on the stove; these reactions can occur over time in closed containers.

Antibacterial properties are produced. Because products of the Maillard reaction produce mutagenic substances, bacteria can be killed. This occurs, for example, when milk sugar (lactose) combines with lysine (or another amino acid) under heat conditions. Killing bacteria can be good, but mutagenic Maillard substances are not.

This causes me to wonder about the cancer-causing potential of unrefrigerated dairy products. First they are irradiated (at a high level - as discussed in a later chapter); then they are exposed to months of warm room and ambient temperatures. Hmm...

Antimutagenic properties can result. Conflicting with the aging and cancer-causing properties above is the production of compounds that are protective against cell damage. Makes no sense? Actually it does. In the Antioxidant chapter this phenomenon is explained under Antioxidant Secret #1 and #3.

The Body Browning Reaction In Your Body
Browning occurs in diabetes mellitus proteins. There are several destructive elements in diabetes; one of them is this non-enzymatic glycosylation. Body and cellular proteins are bonded with sugars, their important properties destroyed. They are then products of this *Body Browning Reaction* (BBR).

Browning can occur in your blood. Glycosylation of hemoglobin, the structure that holds iron and oxygen for your red blood cells, can occur both in certain disease situations and under normal circumstances. There are body mechanisms that take care of this, but they may not be fully operational at certain times.

Cataract formation and connective tissue damage can result. The BBR reaction results in crystals of protein which play a large part in cataract formation. The hardness of the crystals is antithetical to the flexible lens of the eye that is so necessary to see well. This hardness also can be found in stiff connective tissue which often accompanies aging. Excess serotonin is also created by BBR.

Vegetarians and Glycosylation

An interesting note is that vegetarians are often deficient of lysine in their diets because it is a limiting amino acid, and they are known to have fewer of the debilitating diseases that accompany meat eaters.   Could it be that while sacrificing some protein formation due to lack of lysine, they are also saving themselves from the effects of glycosylation?

Antioxidants could be the answer, if we knew which ones to take. Here are a few suggestions.

> **Anti-Aging Food List :**
> **Eat these foods to slow Aging!**
>
> **Brazil Nuts** for selenium.
> (*more than the RDA per nut, about 70ug.)
> **Sunflower seeds** for Vitamin E.
> **Carrots and green veggies like broccoli** for Beta-carotene.
> **Citrus fruits** for Vitamin C, limonene, and hesperidin.
> **Celery** for apigenin.
> **Peppermint, Rosemary** for thymol and menthol
> **Hazelnuts, cashews and olive oil** for monounsaturated fatty acids
> **Whole grains** for fiber (**wheat** for insoluble, **oats/rice** for soluble)
> **Garlic** for alliin and allicin
> **Eggs** for protein and choline

Altzheimers Disease

A low fat diet may help prevent Altzheimers disease. A study indicates that Sweden has the lowest Altzheimers levels anywhere. They eat low fat, fish diets, and not very much beef.

Hormone replacement therapy (estrogen) reduces by 30% the risk of Altzheimers disease.

It is the inhaling of aluminum dust, not cooking with aluminum pans that may be a component of Altzheimers disease.

The Mad Cow Disease connection with Altzheimers is that the identical gooey amyloid plaques that clog the brains of Altzheimers patients are found in victims of Mad Cow Disease. (See BBR discussion above).

Users of Tylenol™ seem to have significantly less Altzheimers disease than users of other over-the-counter pain medications.

Asthma

A daily ingestion of phytoestrogen-containing foods like soy and rye products, may help fend off the effect of dropping estrogen levels that help precipitate an asthma attack. It was found that most asthma attacks in women occur in the place in the menstrual cycle just after estrogen levels nose-dive. (Archives of Internal Medicine, Sept., 1996). So it is my suggestion that a diet rich in these phytoestrogens might help offset the lowered estrogen levels and prevent an asthma attack.

Cancer

Breast Cancer
In "Mammary Cancer Prevention By Regular Garlic and Selenium Enriched Garlic" (Nutrition and Cancer 17:279-286, 1992) it was reported that all members from the Allium family help, in varying degrees, to prevent cancer. This includes shallots, garlic, onion, leek, scallions, and chives. The key is not the amount of selenium, but the level of sulfur compounds like allicin and alliin. The over-the-counter garlic supplement, Kyolic, had a protective effect according to this study.

Other articles have expounded upon garlic's many properties. These include antifungal, antibacterial, antiviral, and anticlotting abilities, as well as the inhibition of the growth of cancer cells *in vitro*.

Strong bones and post-menopausal? You may be more likely to develop breast cancer.

In "ras Gene May Mediate Mammary Cancer Promotion By High Fat", (Nutrition and Cancer 23:283-290, 1995), it was interesting to learn that in order to create optimal tumor growth for the study, 4.7% corn oil was supplied with fish oil to give maximum amounts of linoleic acid (Omega-6). This stimulation of tumor growth appears to work with both breast and prostate cancer cells *in vitro*. Linolenic acid (Omega-3) was suppressive of tumor growth.

Soy products with genistein, daidzein and equol are also inhibitive of tumor growth due to their protein kinase and protease inhibition effect. Inositol phosphate, saponins and phytosterols are three other types of cancer-preventing compounds in soy products. It was found that a low-fat diet (10 -15% of total calories as fat) could inhibit tumor growth as well.

Cereal and fiber intake may be protective against prostate, breast and ovarian cancers. A low caloric intake inhibits promotion of carcinogenesis. This low caloric intake is for omniverous diets; strict vegetarians need not be as concerned with caloric intake.

Aspirin, while protective against colon cancer, appears to do nothing for breast cancer.

Daily soy protein prevents or lessens menopausal symptoms. It is the Genistein, Diadzein, Equol and other phytoestrogens that do the trick.

Fourteen or more alcoholic drinks per week doubles your risk of breast cancer because it may contribute to raised estrogen levels in the blood.

Eat These Foods To Avoid Breast Cancer

Food	Reason
Broccoli	Sulforaphane, Indole-3-carbinol
	Phytoestrogens substitute for bad estrogen
Grapefruit	Soluble carbohydrate, hesperidin
Spinach	Lutein
Soy Foods	Genestein, Diadzein, Equol are some of the
	phytoestrogens that substitute
Fresh Juices	Vitamin B's and C, beta-carotene
Oatmeal	Lowers blood fats
Whole grains,	Insoluble carbohydrates detoxify
Bran	

Ovarian Cancer

It has been reported that ovarian cancer was correlated with high total fat intake (Cancer 58:2363, 1986). This high fat was mostly from meat and milk. Israel has a very high mortality rate from cases of aggressive ovarian cancer, and the disease is most frequent in clusters like the recent large group of post-menopausal New York Jewish women. There is a strong correlation with animal fat and a negative correlation with plant lipids. Ovarian cancer also correlates with obesity in women more than 40% overweight, and in tall women. A low intake of fiber is also suspect in the perpetuation of this type of cancer. An odd, but important note, is that in several studies there was positive correlation with women who used powder after they showered or in their underwear. Avoid using talcum powder in this area.

It should be noted here that even after several well publicized cases, like Gilda Radner and others, most gynecologists are lax in checking for the very few symptoms that present themselves in ovarian cancer. They are also reluctant to discuss it or test for it because it is still a relatively rare cancer. I recently asked a well-known gynecologist / fertility expert how one can know if one has symptoms of ovarian cancer. "Well, if you start to lose a lot of weight..." he began. I interrupted, "Isn't that the end really?" He smiled and said, "Yup" with such a disconcerted air that I was appalled. O.K., what's the moral of this story? Get two opinions and hound your doctor to the point of annoyance until you get the test you feel you need.

Getting Enough Phytoestrogens

You should take in between 30 and 50 milligrams of isoflavones/ phytoestrogens per day. That amount can help prevent breast cancer and osteoporosis, alleviate menopausal symptoms and lower cholesterol. More can be harmful. Do not use supplements.

Below is a list of the phytoestrogen content of some soy products. Remember that phytoestrogens can be found in many plant sources, so vary your source of these potentially beneficial natural compounds.

Soy Sources Of Phytoestrogens

Soy butter 1 Serving (2 Tbsp)	17mg
Soy milk (1 cup)	30mg
Tofu (1/2 cup)	30mg
Tempeh (1/2 cup)	30mg
Soy nuts (1/4 cup)	60mg
Nutlettes cereal (1/4 cup)	61mg

(Nutlettes cereal can be ordered by calling 800-233-3668)

Foods For Women

These foods stimulate estrogen receptors on all of your cells. They each operate in a slightly different way, but all may be useful in the prevention of breast cancer and in offsetting menopausal symptoms. Be aware that the jury is still out on the safety of taking large doses of any type of estrogenic compounds without mediation by other compounds like progestin.

Licorice - Only black licorice qualifies here. Make sure it has actual licorice or licorice root in the candy. Note: Be aware that it may raise your blood pressure temporarily.

Rye Bread - Seeded rye bread contains phytoestrogens that are considered helpful to women.

Tofu / Tempeh / Textured Vegetable Protein - All products with soy protein may be helpful to women due to the isoflavones and phytoestrogens contained within; Equol, Diadzein, and Genistein are three examples of these compounds.

Black Cohosh Tea - Used by the American Indians for years for the various problems of women, it has now been found to have good quantities of phytoestrogenic compounds (Dong Quai, another tea, also has some similar properties)

Grapefruit - Many compounds in grapefruit enhance absorption and effectiveness of compounds like estrogen. If you have a good base of phytoestrogens in your diet, fresh grapefruit will support their functioning.

Broccoli - Sulforaphane and Indole-3-Carbinol are two very important compounds that help prevent breast cancer and other hormonally linked diseases.

Flax - Flax contains one of the highest amounts of alpha-linolenic acid (Omega-3) of any of the seeds of plants tested. Omega-3 works with your blood chemistry properties to help fight cholesterol and disease.

Non-Hodgkin Lymphoma
In "Diet and Risk of Non-Hodgkin Lymphoma in Older Women" (JAMA 275(17), May 1996) it was found that a high meat and/or high fat diet is associated with increased risk of Non-Hodgkins Lymphoma (NHL). NHL represents about 3% of all cancer diagnosed in the U.S. Between 1973 and 1991 the incidence increased 73%. Peyers patches may be a target organ for ingested carcinogens.

This and other studies considered oncogenic viruses, heterocyclic amines, and undegraded proteins and fats. In this study, an amazingly true statement was made. "Food is the largest antigenic challenge facing your immune system." It is so true! We never think about our food as antigenic, but we should. Excess food protein creates hyperstimulation of your immune system. Altered dietary fat alters membrane phospholipid composition.

Prostate Cancer
I always say, if you want prostate cancer, eat fatty food, meats, whole milk, drink alcohol and don't exercise. It happens to be a good recipe for several cancers.

The article "Nutrition and Prostate Cancer" (Nutrition and Cancer 22, 1994) provided a recipe for prevention: reduce total fat, add selenium to your diet, start eating soy products, and reduce the ratio of linoleic (Omega-6) to linolenic (Omega-3) acid in your diet. In other words, eat more linolenic acid (Omega-3). The highest rate of prostate cancer in the world is in the Black American male with a high fat diet. Black Africans have one of the lowest rates. Aggressive prostate cancer is linked to meat, milk and high fat intake, according to this study. The risk increases with high intake of Vitamin A. Vitamin A appeared protective against other cancers in this study (See Antioxidants chapter).

Colon Cancer

Colon cancer correlates with, you guessed it, high total fat consumption and high meat consumption. There are suggestions that coffee (caffeinated), and alcohol contribute to colon cancer. Aspirin has a protective effect. Olive oil and coconut oil did not promote the tumors in a recent study, but corn oil and safflower oil did.

High levels of blood iron may correlate with colon cancer.

For more cancer information, try the New England Journal of Medicine's website (http://www.nejm.org.icic.nci.nih.gov).

Depression

Saint John's Wort may be useful against depression in moderate cases.

Fertility

Women-eat more, exercise less (if you are an aerobics nut or a dieter) and you may see an improvement in fertility as the reproductive hormone leptin begins to rise.

To avoid Pre-Eclampsia and high blood pressure when pregnant, get plenty of calcium (1500 milligrams per day).

Heart Disease/Stroke

New York Times columnist Jane E. Brody recently wrote about the dangers of excess iron in our bodies. In "Potential Dangers of Iron Overload in Rich American Diet", she stated that excess iron "promotes coronary artery disease, fosters latent cancers and infectious organisms". There are bacteria that have iron-loving metabolisms (called siderophores) that will proliferate in a system overloaded with iron. This is one of the reasons that I think zinc supplements work against bacteria. Elemental zinc, offered to the body as Zinc gluconate, competes for the same intestinal sites as iron and thus may reduce the iron stores or bloodstream concentration.

Don't drink wine, drink 10 oz. of purple grape juice (not grape drink) per day. It can reduce your clotting by as much as 40%. Studies at The University of Wisconsin Medical School found it just as effective as aspirin.

Obesity in women (three times normal weight) is a leading risk factor for blood clots in the lungs.

Young girls cannot correct their high cholesterol (above 170) by losing weight.

Depressed mothers give birth to depressed babies. Depression is associated with increased incidence of heart attack.

Lowered cholesterol reduces the risk of stroke.

A man who can't control his anger increases his risk of a heart attack by a factor of three.

Vitamin E may help prevent vasospasms in angina patients according to a recent Japanese study. (More Vitamin E; less pain.)

With respect to heart disease, high insulin levels are as dangerous as high cholesterol, high blood pressure, and sometimes smoking. Eat fewer simple sugars and follow a low fat diet.

The herb Ephedra (Ma Huang) can be very dangerous to your heart if abused.

Suspect a stroke? Ask the victim to smile, lift both arms, and squeeze your hand. Weakness on one side is characteristic of stroke. If the smile is a bit lopsided, the arms don't react the same, or the squeeze is appreciably different, get the victim to an emergency room right away and tell them what you suspect.

Depressed? The risk of stroke is 50% higher; blood platelet activity may trigger clot formation.

Doctors can look for chronic inflammation of the arteries and find heart disease and stroke potential.

Get the amount of potassium in one glass of OJ and one banana every day, and you have a much lower risk of stroke.

MCT (Medium Chain Triglycerides) can raise LDL cholesterol as much as palm kernel oil.

Want to lower high cholesterol and LDL while reducing your risk of heart disease and cancers of the breast and prostate, all with a simple diet change? Get 30 - 50 milligrams per day of the isoflavones in soy products (genistein, diadzein, equol, etc.). How? A quarter cup of roasted soy nuts has 60 milligrams. A Morningstar Farms veggie burger has 8.5 milligrams. Half a cup of tofu or tempeh has 35 milligrams. Call (800) 233-3668 or (800) 445-3350 to get more information on soy protein (Prevention, Jan. 1997).

Donating blood can save you by reducing your iron stores. It can reduce the risk of heart attack by 85%. Too much iron damages your arteries.

Want to lower your blood pressure without drugs? Eat only fruits and vegetables and low fat dairy products for two weeks. You'll be amazed.

Infectious Diseases (Bacteria/Viruses)

Want fewer colds? Get more friends. A strong circle of support is known to strengthen the immune system.

200 milligrams of Vitamin E daily boosts antibody formation and the immune system in the elderly.

The rate of Cholera has shot up to five times its historic low point in the U.S. This may be because more Americans are eating raw seafood and unpeeled fruit in developing countries (Time,1996). Cook all meats and seafoods well, and wash and peel all fruits and vegetables.

If you have chronic bronchitis, you are more likely to have a heart attack.

Smoking-Related Illnesses

Passive smoke near a pregnant woman can cause a baby's lungs to malfunction. The smoke toxins keep oxygen from getting from mother to fetus.

Almost 66% of all deaths attributed to Sudden Infant Death Syndrome (SIDS) may be linked to tobacco smoke, according to British researchers. Even the increased risk of a baby dying from SIDS if brought into a room where smoking has merely occurred, is 800%! (Time™,1996)

Smokers are twice as likely to lose their teeth during their lifetimes as non-smokers.

A Belgian study found that smokers' infants have just as much of a nicotine marker (cotinine) in their urine as the adults.

Ulcers

Your ulcer is not caused by hot foods! It is probably caused by a bacterium called *Helicobacter pylori.* This can be detected by a breath test at your doctor's office. If you are put on the correct antibiotic, the ulcer can disappear!

Miscellany

- Kids who drink 12 oz. of juice per day tend to be fatter and shorter than kids who don't drink as much sweet juice.

- Folic Acid (folate) does not reduce the incidence of neurological birth defects, if the mother-to-be is obese. It only appears to work in thin or average weight pregnant women.

- 200 IU of Vitamin D can slow the progression of osteoarthritis of the knee.

- A good daily dose of calcium lowers the risk of kidney stones. Pass the ice cream please...

- Eggs are good for you! They provide necessary choline for your brain and the most available protein for all of your bodily functions! Have an egg today! (See Reading labels chapter/ Cholesterol section.)

- Don't upset your body clock! You can have immune problems and it just makes you cranky. Varying the time you go to sleep by even a few hours can mess you up for weeks. To reset your body clock, get up at the same time everyday including on the weekend; and go to bed when you're tired.

- Estrogen replacement helps keep your skin elastic (if you're female).

- Grapefruit juice enhances absorption of sedatives, antihistamines, etc.

- Use Organiclean™ The Natural Solution to clean vegetables of dangerous bacteria and viruses. For more information call (888) 834-9274.

- 6 milligrams of Beta-carotene = 1 milligram of Vitamin A.

<u>**Herbal Healing Strategies**</u>

While I do not whole-heartedly recommend all herbal remedies, there are those that do work and those individuals who feel that they must take them. It is for those individuals that I put together this small list. Some of these, like garlic, work well, while others do not. These are traditionally recommended by herbalists for the listed ailments. To treat yourself with any of these herbs, you need specific information which I suggest you <u>only</u> get from people like Varro Tyler (or Jim Duke). Both men have great guides to herbs and usages and vast knowledge about proper dosages. (See Chapter 17 for more information on who you can trust).

Common Herbal Remedies		
Ailment	**Herb That May Help**	**Official Name**
Blood Pressure	Cayenne pepper	*Capsicum sp.*
Blood clots	Garlic	*Allium sativum*
	Ginger	*Zingiber officinale*
	Cloves	*Syzygium aromaticum*
Brain function	Ginko	*Ginko biloba*
	Gotu kola	*Centella asiatica*
Cold	Ma Huang	*Ephedra sinica*
Cholesterol (high)	Garlic	*Allium sativum*
	Niacin in food	Nicotinamide
Heart Troubles	Bird's Eye	*Adonis vernalis*
	Convalotoxin	*Convallaria majalis*
Immune trouble	Mannan	*Aloe vera*
	Ginseng	*Panax ginseng*
Infections	Tea tree oil	*Melaleuca alternifolia*
	Cayenne	*Capsicum sp.*
Melanoma	Betulinic acid	*Ziziphus mauritiana*
	Triterpenoids	*Salvia alba*
Prostate (Enlarged)	Saw Palmetto	*Serenoa repens*
Sleeplessness	Valerian	*Valeriana officinalis*
Stomach upset	Ginger	*Zingiber officinale*
	Mint	*Mentha piperita*

What Foods Can I Eat?

After all of this talk of warfare and news about what chemicals to avoid, here is a concise list of those foods that I think are "Best" for you, and those foods that are "Worst" for you. Remembering that just about all foods can be good or bad depending upon the circumstances, I've also put together a brief list of some common "in-between" foods, with both pros and cons listed.

I don't expect anyone to eat exclusively foods on the "Best" list, and I'm not even advocating that you do so (moderation is the key!). Some of the "Worst" foods might be your favorites, and again, don't worry if you cannot completely eliminate these from your diet. However, I recommend that you review the lists and try to gradually shift your eating patterns to incorporate more of the "Best" foods and fewer of the "Worst". If you can move from "worst" to "in-between", or "in-between" to "best" and maintain these habits for the long haul, you will be doing yourself (and your loved ones) the greatest possible service.

"Best" Foods For You

<u>Whole grains</u> (breads, cereals) - Excellent source of fiber
<u>Skim milk</u> - Low fat, high protein, good calcium source
<u>Lowfat yogurt</u> - Beneficial bacteria, high protein/calcium
<u>Fresh organic fruits/vegetables</u> - Vitamins, minerals, nutraceuticals, fiber
<u>Garlic</u> - High in alliin and allicin
<u>Olive oil</u> - High monounsaturated/low saturated fat
<u>Flax seed oil</u> - High in Omega-3 oil
<u>Soybean products</u> (whole or minimally processed) - Nutraceuticals
<u>Pasta</u> - Low-fat, good carbohydrate source
<u>Rice, Oatmeal</u> - Soluble carbohydrate, good for heart
<u>Nuts</u> - High in protein and minerals
<u>Egg whites</u> - The best protein source
<u>Herbal tea, green tea</u> - Polyphenols and other antioxidants

"In-Between" Foods

<u>Cheese</u> - High in protein, but also high in fat
<u>Whole eggs</u> - Excellent protein source, but high in fat and cholesterol
<u>Poultry</u> - Good protein, lower fat than beef; beware of *Salmonella*/viruses
<u>Fish</u> - Good Omega-3 source, cancer preventative in moderate doses; too much can increase chances of stroke
<u>Black tea</u> - Catechins are anti-cancer; watch for too much caffeine
<u>Coffee</u> - Phenolics in fresh brewed coffee have antioxidant properties; these can be carcinogenic if left to oxidize
<u>Wine</u> - Antioxidant and antimicrobial properties; can be fattening, lower B vitamins, and predispose you to liver problems.

"Worst" Foods For You

Hydrogenated oils (e.g., margarine) - Contain trans fatty acids
Palm oil and coconut oil (and foods which contain these) - High in
    polyunsaturated and saturated fats
Salted, processed, and cured meats (ham, salami, beef jerky) - High in
    fat, salt and nitrates
Beef/Pork - Especially avoid fatty cuts or ground meat.
Fried foods - High in lactones and oxidized fatty acids
Colas - Contain caramel color; high in sugar, too much phosphate
Flavored black tea - Pro-oxidants/carcinogens

Simple substitution suggestions:

Switch oil for butter - to reduce saturated fat
Switch applesauce for oil or butter - reduces total fat
Switch skim milk for whole eggs - reduces saturated fat and
cholesterol

"Best" Manufacturers

Given our hectic schedules, it's not always possible to avoid
processed foods. Following is a list of good responsible food
companies I've found who provide convenience foods that fit into
an overall picture of adequate nutrition. Be aware that there may
be hydrogenated fats in some of these products, so look for the
products without them.

Lightlife Foods, Inc.
P.O. Box 870, Greenfield, MA 01302
(800) 274-6001
Soy based Meat / Hotdogs
Lightlife makes wonderful sausages, hot dogs, and other meatless items. In most cases, you can't tell the difference. I recommend their "Smart Dogs".

Amy's Kitchen, Inc.
P.O. Box 449, Petaluma, CA 94953
Vegetarian Entrees
Amy's Kitchen makes the absolute best frozen vegetarian entrees I have ever had! They're incredible! Made for the couple's young daughter Amy, who was born in 1987, the company prides itself on quality. Choose from pot pie, veggie loaf, shepherd's pie, lasagna, etc. They're all good!

Celentano Bros., Inc.
Verona, NJ 07044
Pasta Entrees
Celentano has always been a company of quality and now they have stepped into the vegetarian/organic foods arena in a big way. I get the feeling that they really care about their customers, and their ravioli and lasagna are wonderful!

Vermont Bread Company
P.O. Box 1217, Brattleboro, VT 05302
Breads
The Vermont Bread Company makes the best whole grain bread around! They use little fat, and healthy whole grains in most of their breads. Whole grains are not as common in bread as you might think; many manufacturers use the words "stoneground", "wheat", "unbleached", and "enriched" to entice the public to purchase their breads. Once again, read the labels. If there's lots

of junk in the bread, if it doesn't actually say whole wheat (or other grain), or if you see partially hydrogenated oils; run, don't walk, to the nearest healthy loaf of bread. The texture will be different too. Good breads are roughly grained and textured and heavy. If your bread is smooth, soft and light, you may be paying for less than you should be getting.

Morningstar Farms
Worthington Foods, Worthington, OH 43085
Morningstar Farms breakfast links are the closest tasting and textured to real sausage that anyone is likely to get. I have fooled a number of people with them. Of course I told them later that what they were eating was actually better for them than the real thing, but the looks of surprise were fun. I break them up for use in meated recipes as well.

Green Giant™/Pillsbury Company
2866 Pillsbury Center, Minneapolis, MN 55402-1464
(800) 998-9996
Imitation Hamburger
Italian patties and other varieties of hamburger are the mainstay so far of this branch of Green Giant. The hamburgers are nicely flavored and we all enjoy them, but you will not be fooled into thinking that these are real meat, which in many ways is a probably a good thing; you should know what you're eating.

There are vegans who say that imitating meat products defeats the whole purpose of living without them. Here I must break rank with the party line because some people who otherwise would never consider vegetarianism except after a heart attack or discovery of cancer or diabetes, will try these ersatz meat products. And that's a good outcome.

Tree Tavern Pizza
Pizza (Fresh or Frozen)
The frozen pizza with the least oil and gunk in it is Tree Tavern.
Look for partially hydrogenated oils or high fructose corn syrup in
the other brands

Muir Glen Organic Sauces
P.O. Box 1498, Sacramento, CA 95812
Tomato Sauce
They make several tasty sauces which don't have added oils or
high fructose corn syrup as filler. Look for partially hydrogenated
oils or high fructose corn syrup in the other brands.

Breakfast Cereals
Familia™ - Wholesome ingredients and a choice of sugared or
non-sugared cereal provides a good, healthy breakfast, but also a
fattening one.

Quaker™ Oatmeal - Whole Oats are better than Quick Quaker
Oats as a whole food, but it may be more heart beneficial to get the
already broken oats for ease of absorption of the complex
carbohydrates that lower cholesterol.

Cheerios™ - Although the formula was changed a couple of years
ago to have modified food starch instead of some of the oat
content, they still are low in fat, sugar and salt. I wish they still
had that old Cheerios™ oat taste though...Other types of
Cheerios™ (Honey Nut, Multigrain, etc.) contain partially
hydrogenated fats and oils as well.

Raisin Bran - Whether Post™ or Kellogg™, it really makes little
difference. The insoluble fiber helps aid digestion, and if that's
what you need, eat this cereal. It also is loaded with sugar and

vitamins, of which you absorb virtually none. The vitamins are lost as you might suspect because of the high fiber content. But it is good to eat raisin bran if you don't get enough vegetables or fruits; at least you're getting necessary insoluble fiber.

Snyder's Pretzels
Pretzels
Pretzels are an excellent alternative to fried snack foods like potato chips and tortilla chips. Snyder's pretzels have the most wholesome ingredients I've found, and there are fat-free and salt-free varieties. Avoid pretzel varieties with added flavorings, which can make them as bad as chips.

<u>Do Not Eat</u>

Store brands
It is better not to eat boxed or canned versions of your favorite foods that are store-brand foods. Although the quality is said to be the same as the name brand, it seldom is. The store-brand paper goods will save you money though.

Foreign produce
There are too many pesticides, heavy metals and unsanitary conditions to be able to recommend foreign produce. Ask at your market where the produce comes from before you buy it. Pesticides which are banned in the U.S. are being manufactured and sold to third world countries and the pesticides return to us on produce.

Where does your produce come from? According to a recent article in The Newark Star Ledger (June 1997), "...Produce has largely been exempted from country-of-origin labeling laws." Representative Sonny Bono was sponsoring a bill to change that.

Foods With Artificial Color In Them
These compounds will oxidize your cells, giving you cancer potential.

Foods With Lots Of Saturated Or Polyunsaturated Fat
Saturated fat ruins your cells' ability to communicate with one another, and can accelerate fatty tissue cancers.

Too Much Meat
Meat is hard on the digestive system. Saturated fat can harden and clog arteries. And beef contains toxins, hormones and pesticides, not to mention the possibility of Mad Cow Disease.

Chapter 17
THE EXPERTS

After listening to a prominent talk show queen discuss her "Nutritionist" and the odd things that went on in her "sessions," I began to realize that it doesn't matter how famous or wealthy you are, you can still be taken in by the wiles of a charlatan. Nutritionists, as defined in Chapter 1, are by nature an ill-defined lot anyway. Anyone who wants to, can hang out a shingle and call themselves a nutritionist.

If you've gotten this far, you certainly appreciate the enormous amount of nutritional information there is to sift through. And more research is being done all the time, so you can expect the picture to become even more complicated. You need to be careful about who you select to guide you through the maze that is nutrition. I have listed some people I believe are credible in their respective fields. It is not all-inclusive; there are some very good people who I have not encountered enough to recommend, and there are people I have deliberately left off.

Who can you trust, and for what?

Take Advice From

Andrew Weil
Author of the watershed guide to renewed health, "Spontaneous Healing" (1996), he hits the nail on the head when it comes to classical medical training. It is a "must read." Several of his colleagues criticize him for attempting to undermine traditional

medical treatment, but it is an unfair and uneducated position to take. While some nutrient and herbal ideas (like Ayurvedic) are far afield from what I might advocate, "Spontaneous Healing" is a medical "Emperor's New Clothes". Physicians have played God for too long.

Isadore Rosenfeld
He writes credibly about herbs and alternative healing in his latest book, <u>The Guide To Alternative Medicine</u> and explains what works and why. He is also a regular health commentator on a major television network.

Tim Johnson
A good scientific examination of the evidence presented is what he gives his listeners during his television reports. He presents credible findings and looks at them with a scientist's critical eye. He is not your average MD.

Dean Ornish
He writes and speaks credibly about health and heart issues. I recommend his books and lectures. On this topic for years before it became a *cause celebre*, he can take some credit for helping to propel healthy eating and exercise as preventative medicine into the spotlight.

Neal Barnard
President of Physicians Committee For Responsible Medicine, he is concerned with our great consumption of fatty meats, dairy products, empty calories and our lack of exercise. While there is an agenda to his talks, his advice is usually sound and credible. I can recommend his books and lectures.

Varro Tyler

Professor Emeritus of Pharmocognosy at Purdue University, he knows vast amounts about the safety and efficacy of herbal and natural treatments for disease. He is currently writing for Prevention™ Magazine.

James Duke

Considered a world authority on the medicinal uses for botanicals and herbs, he started out as a botanist fascinated by folklore surrounding the use of herbal pharmaceuticals. He understands the chemistry of herbs and their relation to currently accepted pharmaceutical preparations. His latest book, The Green Pharmacy, is a must for anyone interested in herbs and their safe and effective usage.

Covert Bailey

Author of Smart Eating, he expunges the myths about diet and exercise. His good common sense suggestions include exercising more, and eating fruits and vegetables to lose weight.

Jane Brody

An excellent columnist for the New York Times, she can distill a nutrition or health issue to comprehensibility without losing the good scientific content. Read her column. Her books The Book of Health and Nutrition are the ones I prefer.

Richard Simmons

He truly cares about the overweight and has done an amazing amount of good on their behalf. Use his tapes and books for motivation and his great low fat recipes. Try his new Sweetie Pie and Farewell To Fat cookbooks and his Sweatin' tapes.

Prevention™ Magazine
Credible advice and hints about everything from diet and exercise
to sex and heart disease, a Prevention™ subscription is a must in
your healthy home.

Jean Carper
Wonderful reports in Parade magazine were how I first
encountered the writings of Jean Carper. She is also the author of
many books that are clearly written and accessible to anyone. It is
such an important service to deliver nutritional information without
watering down content. She does this well.

Other people you can trust to bring you the most current
information include:

- Carolyn O'Neil (CNN)
- Walter Willett (Harvard University)
- Paul Lachance (Rutgers University/Nutraceutical Institute)
- Michael Guillen (TV correspondent)
- Max Gomez, (NBC News)
- Herbert Pierson (Author of The Diet-Cancer Link)
- Victor Herbert (Author of Total Nutrition)

Be Cautious With Advice From

Your Doctor
He may be clueless. While Hippocrates himself recognized a
connection between nutrition and health (the first case was a
Vitamin A deficiency), 78% of American medical schools still do
not require doctors to take a nutrition course. Of the ones that do,
most require only one such course. Most doctors know very little
about nutrition, in spite of what they would like you to think. If
you are interested in your health and long life, you need to become

an expert in nutrition yourself. One or two books (from the credible people listed above) and you will have exceeded the total knowledge your doctor probably has about nutrition. It's not his fault, really. American medical schools are so hung up on traditional medicine that they have ignored anything else, to the detriment of their patients.

I personally know of physicians who have advocated that their pregnant patients start drinking alcohol to "calm their nerves". Guess they haven't heard about fetal alcohol syndrome. One doctor ordered his pregnant patient to stop drinking orange juice because "it's fattening." We have to assume that he's not aware of folic acid deficiencies, sources of folic acid, or the serious neural tube defects that a fetus can have if the mother doesn't get enough. Most physicians do not know what to eat or what to avoid, or why. It hasn't been a priority until recently.

And they go way too far making diagnoses for you! No one can really give you your risk of getting cancer after exposure to a carcinogenic substance. Your family physician (or even an oncologist) might tell you, "Don't be silly, no one ever gets cancer from one exposure" or he/she might have said to you or someone dear to you, "I'm sorry, but you have less than a year to live." The doctor does not have enough knowledge to make either of these calls, yet is willing to do it all the time! I would say that's the ultimate in chutzpah! Do not let your physician tell you how long you will live! He does not know! If you do take the doctor's word for it, your life will only be as long as he has said. Below is the classic example of such a self-fulfilling prophesy.

Your medical doctors are specialists in tracking the development of the different stages of cancer, specialists in surgery, treatments and aware of certain statistics surrounding cancers that they work with. If the average person dies within a year, will you? Maybe, maybe not. But <u>the answer lies within you, not the doctor</u>. You can decide what to do and how to do it. Look at AIDS patients, condemned to all die within two years in the early 1980's. Now many of them live well past 10 years, with no major infections! Why? It is not just an immune resistance to the strain they got; no, it is a will to live, to continue.

What does this all mean? It means that nothing is written in stone, and individual differences in many aspects from immune functioning to your focus in life can change your outcome. Events occurring simultaneously with the development of disease or cancer can accelerate the process or serve to decelerate it. Your attitude toward the physician as all-knowing, second only to God, will send you right down the path to his/her diagnosis. You'll have what he/she says you'll have and you'll die when you're told you will. If you act this way, you'd better find an optimist for a doctor or you're in big trouble! I heard the following story several years ago (possibly from Dr. Bernie Siegel); it is worth sharing.

A hypochondriac woman was admitted to a hospital, complaining of aches and pains, but the doctors could find nothing wrong with her. She was forever hounding the medical staff, talking about how near death she might be if they didn't find her problem. Finally one nurse found a tiny infection on her foot. The nurse wrote "TC" on her chart for "Toe Carbuncle" and a release date for her. In the habit of checking her chart at the end of the bed after each visit, she was shocked! "I'm a Terminal Case! I knew it! And they've given me only two weeks to live!" Amazingly she relaxed after the diagnosis and became a better patient. Unfortunately, she believed what she thought was on the chart and up and died on the date specified. Talk about cooperative! Many of us rely heavily on the opinion of one physician and are cooperative patients. Do not be a cooperative patient. It could ruin your life!

If you are concerned about a food or nutrient interaction, do not ask your physician, ask a good pharmacist or nutritionist.

Non-MD Doctors
While I have blasted away at traditional medical doctors (those with an M.D.), there are others who call themselves "doctors" who may have even less credibility in some cases. These are Doctors of Osteopathy (D.O.) and Doctors of Chiropractic (D.C.). The training and educational requirements for the recipients of these degrees are generally less stringent than for M.D.s. Osteopaths may have more holistic training, though.

A chiropractor has even less traditional medical training and bases his practice on the alignment of your spinal column. This may or may not have more than a little scientific credibility. Unfortunately, for the many sincere and careful chiropractic doctors out there, there are many more charlatans than are found in traditional medicine because the field is less regulated. And the traditional medical practices are wary of recognizing them as helpful for that reason and the fact that some poor scientific concepts are perpetuated by such individuals.

There are always going to be individuals who try to narrow you down to some organ or type. If you go with an ailment to a specific sort of doctor, you'll hear different things. The cardiologist wants to listen to your heart, the gastroenterologist (if he's a good one) asks, "What's going on in your life?", the surgeon's answer always is, "Let's remove it", while the chiropractor says, "Let's crack your back a little", and the proctologist always says, "Bend over".

Hospital Dieticians
I have taught a number of dieticians in my years of teaching Nutrition and Microbiology, and I caution you, once again, to find

your own way through the nutritional maze. My 95-year old grandmother, who was just about completely vegetarian by the time she had her first heart attack, awoke on the morning after her myocardial infarction to SAUSAGE, EGGS, and toast with BUTTER! She was later served STEAK by the hospital nutrition staff for dinner! Gee, that's just the thing for the heart attack patient who has recently started eating mostly vegetables! I was horrified! But this is not an isolated case; rather it is the norm, with many young dieticians being taught antiquated nutritional standards.

"There are a million excuses, ranging from cost to the inability of cooks to prepare healthful food..." says Marion Nestle, Professor of Nutrition and Food Studies at New York University, in a recent interview for Leslie Dickstein in Self magazine. She added, though, "But in a hospital where someone cares about it, the problems get solved."

Public Interest Groups
Public interest groups are important for alerting the consumer about certain food facts that they might otherwise not have known. The problem comes when these groups grab at one study with questionable data gathering and the study is treated like words that fell from the lips of God. Consumers don't ever realize a study is faulty; they never get to judge for themselves. They must trust such groups and reporters. So there are people who've just switched to the current "good" food without any other corroboration, just a TV report or a small article in the newspaper.

The tendency of public interest groups to make inflammatory and sometimes even untrue "scientific" pronouncements is dangerous. The recent suggestion, brought forth by one such group, that a roast beef sandwich is better for you and less fattening than a tuna fish sandwich is ludicrous. Why? First, who made the sandwiches? Some all-you-can-eat diner? No one I know makes more fattening tuna sandwiches than roast beef ones. Did they both have mayonnaise, as they normally do? Many people get roast beef sandwiches with mayonnaise; tuna is made with mayonnaise. Were they the same exact weight? If both meat quantities were identical, and the condiments were equal, the tuna sandwich would probably be less fatty than the roast beef one. Tuna is also lower in saturated fat and higher in those fatty acids we are supposed to ingest, like Omega-3 (alpha-Linolenic). Take every report with a grain of salt until you hear it from a credible source. The people who are responsible for data interpretation in these groups are reporters, not scientists.

People Who Suggest Protein or Carbohydrate-Only Diets
The desire to sell books can overwhelm the regard for patient health. While such diets really can work, they are very dangerous to be on for a long time. Protein-only diets can precipitate kidney problems if abused. High protein can interfere with magnesium and calcium levels as well. Carbohydrate-only diets can create immune troubles, healing problems and mineral absorption issues.

These diets may occasionally be prescribed - by competent professionals - for very specific conditions, and under strict supervision. If your doctor is putting every other patient in his office on one of these diets, the red alert should go off in your head.

The Health Food Store Clerk or Owner
File this advice under the category of "What possible motivation could I have?" and take it with a grain of salt. While their recommendations could be true, there is often no science or credible basis for "factual" statements and you are taking a chance using their advice.

People Selling Pills
Back in the days of the wild west, charlatans would travel from one
backwater town to the next, hawking "magic elixirs" guaranteed to
cure everything but the weather. Today, their descendants can still
be seen on TV or in the magazines. They tout the latest
"nutritional breakthroughs". And as fate would have it, they just
happen to have that magic elixir available for $19.95 (plus
shipping & handling). What a remarkable coincidence!

Let's all repeat the mantra. Nutrition is not about pills. Nutrition
is about foods. Whole, wholesome, healthy foods. If you really
believe that a certain compound is good for you, find a food rich in
the substance and eat more of it. Take supplements only when
absolutely necessary, and in moderation.

People Who Stray From Their Field
There is a tendency, when one puts pen to paper, to offer
philosophy, as I do in this book, along with facts. Often the line
between the two can be blurred if the practitioner of some unusual
healing practice is also a physician. Use sources for their advice in
fields in which they have credentials, not always in fields that are
unrelated.

Linus Pauling was a Nobel laureate in his chosen field,
Biochemistry, and he later began advocating unusual nutritional
regimens. These regimens went from useless to potentially
harmful with the advocation of 10,000 milligrams of Vitamin C
every day. Vitamin C is very important, but at that level you will
lose electrolytes due to heavy bouts of diarrhea. You also risk
running short on other nutrients including Vitamin B-12, which is
depleted by large doses of Vitamin C.

One-Nutrient Charlies

> DHEA will make you younger!
> BEE POLLEN made my wife fall in love with me!
> MELATONIN can wax your car for you too!

The claims get wilder and wilder all the time! There is no single nutrient or natural supplement that it makes sense to take all the time, or in pill form. None. These "One Nutrient Charlies" are out to sell books, supplements, or both. And while no nutritionist worth his/her salt will tell you that you get the RDA of vitamins and minerals just from food, they will only recommend supplements on a limited basis, like taking Centrum™ every three days or so. Because **you don't need the RDA every day**! In the U.S. we are rarely seriously deficit of any one nutrient, so we should not need to tinker with our body chemistry on a daily basis.

Which Studies Can You Trust?

Retrospective Studies
Retrospective studies look at current human health and disease statistics in comparison with past nutritional habits. These studies can examine the last two weeks worth of eating and look at the change in chemicals in the bloodstream, or they can look at the past ten years of intake and decide which factors contributed to your current health status. Retrospective studies are hampered by the fact that human memory is imperfect, and even the most tireless researchers and most extensive studies cannot account for everything that happened in the past. They do provide us with a very good basis for generalizing about food groups we should favor, and basic dietary guidelines.

Prospective Studies

Prospective studies look, as the name implies, forward through current human consumption to future effects. They are a slight improvement over Retrospective studies because there is greater control over consumption into the future. Patients can be asked to eat at certain times of the day, eat only certain foods, or report on practices that may affect results. They can then be measured before during and after to see any weight changes, blood or urine changes, etc. The researcher has more leeway to construct controlled studies.

Balance Studies

Balance studies look at the amount of a nutrient going into the human body versus that which leaves. Everything can be measured, including sweat, saliva, urine, blood or feces, to determine the useable amount of a nutrient. This gives us one of the most important tools for assessing **Bioavailability**, an important measure of how much of a nutrient is available to you after you ingest it.

Bacterial Studies

The Ames Test, developed by Dr. Bruce Ames, correlates up to 90% with compounds later found to cause cancer. The Ames test looks at the ability of the given chemical to mutate or alter the organism or its DNA in some deleterious way. It works like a charm. All that is needed is to get FDA approval to use this and other similar studies in place of almost useless animal studies. Talk to your local Congressman. They will actually do something if you write to them. Very few people take the time to put pen to paper and get involved. Just do it.

Which Studies Can You Seldom Trust?

I have worked as a biologist for the last 15 years. I have worked with and tested animals throughout this time (rabbits, mice, horses, rats). I have come to the following conclusion: testing for cancer in laboratory animals is very ineffective. Do not believe all of these tests when you hear about the results. Take everything with a grain of salt.

Why Are These Tests Less Than Credible?

Amounts of chemicals being tested are too high to ever compare to human data or consumption. The saccharin and cyclamate tests were so ridiculously over-the-top they were lampooned at every turn. Even the old comedy show Fernwood Tonight ™ did an "experiment" to prove that the wearing of leisure suits caused cancer, reducing the credibility of such studies even more.

Does animal research compare the lifetime dose of humans adequately with the shortened lives of experimental animals? Are they allowed to live their lives out in groups or families before we assess the damage done to them by whatever chemical we're using on them, like humans do?

The "time factor" is *accelerated* by using higher doses of experimental drugs. This makes little sense, except to show the great impatience of the research community for quick easy data. You cannot compare the huge doses given a rat with the amount and effect of much less of a chemical dose given to a human being over a much longer time period.

Lots of things happen in the 70+ year typical lifespan of a human being that don't happen to a caged rat. The human being has hope, successes, love of another of his species, offspring. The experimental rat has nothing. The human being has access to lots of information that might help him avoid disease. The rat has nothing. These differences are real and change the way disease accelerates.

If a human being lived like the rat, hopeless, isolated from his own species, in constant fear, in constant pain---Gee, I wonder what would happen. Of course the human would develop some debilitating disease like cancer or some chronic illness. It's almost a given. If an experiment is to have credibility, plans need to be made to allow the animal to live out its entire life span comfortably, in a grouping of others of its own species. At least this way we would know the true effects on the life of laboratory animals. Only then could we make correlations, if speculatively, with human effects.

Often there is no analog to human reaction as in the thalidomide disaster, where every type of animal was tested including dogs and thalidomide was determined safe for expectant mothers. The result was puppies that were fine, but human babies born without arms or legs or both. DES (Diethylstilbesterol) is another example of a drug that was found to be safe in animals, but caused cancer in the offspring of women who used it. Aspirin kills cats, but is sometimes O.K. in dogs and humans...Oops! Penicillin kills guinea pigs, but it's O.K. for humans. Another error! When you are sick, you don't send your spouse to the doctor, do you? I don't need to know how something affects guinea pigs, I need to know how it affects humans!

There are dozens of ways to experiment on humans without causing harm. Computer models using previous data and carefully harvested current numbers would yield better results. Epidemiological studies would display cancer and disease demographics. *In vitro* human cells could be tested using a test similar to the Ames Test mentioned previously. Non-invasive techniques on volunteers, or even voluntary invasive tests like testing a new AIDS vaccine on the 50 doctors who are willing to have it tested on themselves in order to circumvent arcane regulations, would be an improvement on the current situation.

Isolated organs and cells don't tell the whole story! When you do something to an animal and then remove its liver to see what happened, you are trying to assess a physiological change with gross anatomy. When you perfuse (run liquid through) the same liver to see its functioning, it doesn't work like it would inside an animal either. No animal organ or cell can be studied in isolation and give you any real human biochemical answers, just gross anatomical ones. Why does no one get this? All the wasted time and money in research labs across the country is amazing.

Then there is the thought, "O.K., well, I'll just tie the animal down and do gastric lavage (run liquid through the animal for days, weeks, or years). That'll give me the answers to <u>human disease</u>." No, it won't! Does it occur to these scientists that I'm never going to have my arms and legs taped down (I hope), have a hole cut in my stomach, a tube inserted, and days of unending pain as colas or experimental fats are poured through me? No, any disease or changes I get will be <u>from eating a normal amount of the stuff</u> over time. These badly designed experiments just don't cut it!

Much of the work has already been done! Few scientists are willing to trust someone else's work and so, in some cases, experiments are <u>repeated</u> by different researchers. In a few instances this is necessary. But in most cases, the work is more repetitive than follow-on, and is scientifically unnecessary. All one has to do is really search through the literature, both chemical and biological, to look for connections to what one wants to study. It is easier, unfortunately, just to do a quick search and use whatever papers support your idea.

Follow-on experiments that determine the validity of spurious research are often, themselves, poorly designed as well. It is a shame, but researchers working with animals are often ignorant about correct methods of scientific studies, like replicates and controls and the need to look at other factors like living conditions. They also are ignoring causal relationships between other factors besides the one they're looking at and disease. More meta-analysis of data should be considered up front during experimental design.

Similar chemicals have already been looked at! In many cases, there are analogs to chemicals that are unnecessarily studied. If a type of chemical has been studied, there should be a national database that allows access to this information. Assumptions could be made about its cancer-causing capabilities and less expensive research would be needed. These assumptions would have to err on the negative side; for example, if a chemical were to be found to cause cancer in a fairly controlled study, then similar chemicals should be branded as potential cancer-causers. "Similarities" would be determined by comparison to exact chemical formulas in such a database. Adjuvants, routes of administration, chemical complexities, and other factors about the patient would need to be considered as well, when setting up this database.

Despite the gnashing of teeth and wailing of researchers everywhere, there is good science in looking at chemical predictability by similar structure. It's just that no one has a vested interest in ending wasteful research. Such a database would only serve the public and prevent unnecessary studies. "Where's the money in that?" would be the hue and cry of animal scientists at pharmaceutical and laboratory-based companies everywhere.

The lack of such organized information is the reason there are "Orphan drugs"; drugs desperately needed by dying patients. These patients have to wait months or years until a certain number of animals are butchered before the safety of the drug can be determined. **But searching such a database and making safe assumptions would take minutes!** You could have your safety risks analyzed immediately. All that would be needed is testing of the patients blood, a physical, a nutritional analysis; and voila, we'd have a personally tailored analysis of whether a drug would pose "X %" of risk, and to whom. Then it would be the doctor and patient's choice. Isn't there a biochemist out there who knows enough about his/her subject to set this up?

Stress. It is never considered a factor in the induction of disease in animals, but always looked at in humans. Venerable physicians like Dr. Bernie Siegel, the author of "Love, Medicine, and Miracles" (an excellent resource) know that stress is important in the creation of human disease. It is felt that we almost create our own cancers. This is not blaming the victim. This asks, "What else is going on in your life? Are you under stress? Do you believe in God?", etc. Dr. Siegel has said that you can almost determine the outcome of a given cancer or surgery by the amount of love, prayer and will surrounding a patient. He started his research simply, by whispering into the ears of comatose, post-surgical or dying patients. He whispered words of hope and confidence in their recovery. The results were amazing. Those he whispered to did much better than control subjects.

We are animals. We tie down other animals and cut them without anaesthesia. We shove them around, inject them, cut out their organs while they are living - to see what happens. Could this create STRESS? I wonder. How smart do we have to be to see that there is a connection between the stress an animal in an experiment is under and the induction of cancer? Even those in the beef slaughter industry know that stress right before slaughter ruins and changes the quality of the meat! How many Ph.D.s or M.D.s with no common sense will it take before we realize that we've been harming the public and wasting everybody's time with many of these useless efforts?

I am a scientist with credentials. I believe in science. Don't misunderstand me. There are good, credible, hard-working scientists that often labor in obscurity. But what I'm telling you is the ugly truth about the bad studies. I've seen what some of this bad science does to torment the animals. Many of these studies are poorly designed as well. In some studies the only merit the research has is that it is working (in some bizarre unscientific way) on the "cause of the day". Whatever the major topic in the public health realm, we know that some unscrupulous scientist will switch his research to it to get the big money. Concern for controls, replicates, credibility and even the environment of the animal subjects is secondary to the big paycheck.

The review process for the merits of these studies should include a wider circle of members of the educated public, not old cronies patting one another on the back and letting any old project get funded just because it is the prevailing issue of the day. This is dangerous to the public health and welfare. The animal "stress" issue alone negates the "scientific" result in many studies, because the heavy amount of stress alone could have been what induced cancer in the animals. Can any of my colleagues prove otherwise? No, they cannot. Unless animals are treated in a truly humane way that supports a life with less stress (not just using the minimal codes that were forced on researchers a few years ago), we can trust few of these studies. Even the EPA agrees, stating in the

Federal Register in 1991, "There are inherent uncertainties in quantitative risk assessment because, among other things, of the necessity of relying on data from animal studies to predict human risk."

Chapter 18
HEALTH TIPS FOR
A DISEASE-FREE LIFE

1.   Read All Labels.

Always read labels! How else will you know what you are ingesting? It is a very simple task, and worthwhile.

In Chapter 3, we looked at a typical nutritional label. You may want to look at that chapter again, now that we have discussed the various nutritional components in detail.

2.   Do not exceed 30 grams of fat per day, but never go less than 10 grams per day.

Try to eat mostly monounsaturated fats. Minimize saturated fats, and eat only those polyunsaturated fats that are essential (Linoleic, Linolenic, Arachidonic). Avoid too much linoleic acid (Omega-6) fatty acid. Try to get more alpha-linolenic acid (Omega-3). Get this fat from foods, not in pills. See Chapter 6 for more information on fats.

Eat a maximum of 30 grams of total fat per day. My suggestion is, shoot for 20 grams and miss. If you exceed this fat intake on a regular basis, you will get fat.

3.   Eat 40 - 50 grams of protein per day.

Use varied sources of amino acids obtained from whole foods, not supplements. If you are a vegetarian, try to get enough of the amino acids lysine and methionine.

As we discussed in Chapter 7, do not overdo it with protein; it can cause you serious problems.

4.   . Eat at least 100-125 grams of carbohydrate daily.

Eat mostly complex carbohydrates and some simple ones. Eat less refined sugar; this includes white, brown, dark brown, turbinado, and fructose sugars. If you need sugar, try to get it from fruit. Carbohydrates are discussed in detail in Chapter 8.

5.   Avoid hydrogenated fats.

Hydrogenated and partially hydrogenated fats are in virtually everything! Just try and avoid it if you eat processed foods! Even some "good" organic, vegetarian frozen entrees have it! Insist that your grocer carry alternate foods that do not have partially hydrogenated fats in them.

One of the most popular chocolate wafer cookies has always had LARD in it as well as partially hydrogenated fat. See if you can find it in the cookie aisle at your supermarket.

6.   Avoid artificial colors.

This includes soda, cookies and anything that has color artificially added to it. Carmel coloring has been known for 20 years to cause cancer, but it's still in everything! Many of the other dyes (Red, Blue, Yellow tartrazine) are under-regulated in your food because the manufacturers say to the FDA, "Who's gonna eat that much snack food anyway? There's very little dye per serving..." And they get away with it.

Red dye #2 has an interesting history. The food scientists in the U.S. have declared it unsafe so we have had it removed from any food that falls under that legislation (although you can still find it in inexpensive candy if you look for it).

Canada and all of Europe have relied on their educated scientists and their data suggest that Red dye #2 is O.K.; it's Red dye #40 that causes cancer! Here in the U.S. we use liberal amounts of Red dye #40! This is one of the reasons I suggest avoiding dyes altogether. All of this animal testing is conflicting and meaningless. Just stay away from dyes in general.

7.   Throw out all food on the "For Sale Until" date.

This may sound a little over the top, but it is very important. Sometimes the manufacturer will stretch the time a little, exposing you to fungus, bacteria, epoxides and other cancer-causing compounds. Get rid of your old food!

8.   Don't scrape mold off cheese.

How many times have you scraped mold off cheese to serve or eat it? Well, don't do it again! Mold has Hyphae, or invisible tentacles, that reach throughout the entire cheese. These hyphae are extensions of the mold you cut off and can generate toxins or dangerous spoilage in other parts of the cheese.

9.   Get rid of old bread.

While bread is not subject to bacterial decay, all sorts of molds can and do grow invisibly inside! Bread, rolls, bagels and other leavened products all have the potential to carry toxins that food scientists have not found that are dangerous and cancer-causing! Think about *aflatoxin*, the extremely powerful cancer-causing fungal product found in corn and peanuts. It would not be any fun to find out that the bread you always reheated in the microwave when it got stale was what gave you cancer.

10.   Eat foods whose dishes you can clean effectively with water.

Sounds unusual? Not really. If the food you eat requires lots of detergent to get off the pans and plates, you're eating way too much fat or sugary/fat combinations of foods. If you can rinse your plate clean easily with water (Always use very hot water and soap to clean your dishes, regardless!), then you are probably eating good combinations of lower fat foods.

It is absolutely imperative that you clean dishes in water so hot it would burn you without thick rubber gloves. Otherwise, you will leave bacteria and viruses alive on your plates and cups even after they're dried and put away. Rinse dishes with clean tap water as many times as you can stand it. To get rid of absolutely everything, 20 rinses is suggested. I know that's way over the top for the average dishwasher, but I thought you'd like the microbial facts here.

Load your dishwasher so that you will not touch the eating surfaces of your plates, cups, bowls and utensils when unloading. Never pick up cups or bowls with your fingers inside them. You are putting all of your living hand germs (bacteria, fungi, viruses) on surfaces where they'll happily grow. <u>Always</u> put forks, knives, and spoons into the dishwasher upside-down so you can remove them without grasping the eating surface.

11.   Go organic.

Does it make a difference? Absolutely! The fewer man-made pesticides you ingest over a lifetime, the better off you are. Pesticides are systemic in some vegetables and fruits like peaches. This means that they cannot be removed just by washing the fruit. And sometimes they change into much more serious chemical compounds!

Remember the Alar scare? Farmers considered it harmless to use on their apples because "no one eats that many" apples anyway. It was then pointed out that <u>children</u> eat lots of fruit and fruit juices. This additional intake, combined with children's size and stage of development, made them much more vulnerable than adults to the effects of foreign chemicals in the food.

The denouement was that Alar changed into a component of rocket fuel upon heating; a molecule called UDMH (apple juice is made by heating apple slurry). The ensuing hue and cry removed Alar from standard use and it is now used only in isolated cases.

So the world is safe. Not so fast - hundreds of other pesticides are going into your apples and other produce! One of the biggest problems with pesticide use today is that there are literally hundreds of pesticides out there that are put into use in the U.S. <u>without testing</u>! Think about that! We are being exposed to many foreign chemicals in our produce without our permission. This has always annoyed me. There's no denying that there are unusual compounds created after the processing of foods sprayed with certain pesticides.

What to do? Go Organic! Look for the NOFA label. It stands for Northeast Organic Farmers Association. Each state has a chapter. In California, it's COFA. Here in New Jersey, it's NOFA-NJ. It's getting easier to find organically-grown produce all the time. If your grocers don't stock it, urge them to start.

12.   Stay out of the sun.

There are two types of ultraviolet (UV) rays to watch out for. UVB rays will build up your chances for sunburn and cancer; UVA rays will ravage and age your skin. And one bad sunburn puts you in the high-risk group for one of the deadliest skin cancers, malignant melanoma. There are other sun-given cancers like the basal cell carcinoma that former President Ronald Reagan had removed from his nose, but melanoma is the most worrisome.

Your doctor might not know what melanoma looks like (not too many GPs do), he/she might worry about being wrong if he/she suspects it, and neither you or your doctor might see it if it's between your toes or hidden on your back. This brings me to a very important part of keeping free of cancer.

13.   Read everything and do self-examinations.

There are so many people who are waiting to give you pamphlets and show you how to do self exams for breast, testicular, colon, and other cancers, you'll probably run into one within the week. There are yearly and monthly clinics in every place from the mall to the doctor's office. The best information comes from the

American Cancer Society. They'll explain the risks of certain types of diets, smoking, and so on.

14.   Keep an immaculate kitchen and bathroom.

This is not just for looks. Anyone can straighten a room to look clean; you need to use lots of soap and water to clean your counters and food serving and preparation surfaces. They should be as close to sterile and antimicrobial as you can safely get. This doesn't mean using dangerous chemicals in order to sanitize.

15.   No pesticides in the house!

And don't use roach, ant, or bug spray! These noxious chemicals linger for years in your dust and air, exposing you to cancer-causing chemicals and toxins. Got bugs? Starve them out! Keep your kitchen so air tight and clean, they simply move away!

16.   Compartmentalize your kitchen.

Many foodborne illnesses are caused by our own inattention to microbial details. A simple way to minimize problems is to keep "floor" items on the floor and "counter" items on the counter! If you put shoes, wastebaskets, mops, grocery bags or other items that have been on dirty floors onto or above your counter surface, you have contaminated your counters with countless bacteria (including the organism that causes Botulism!) and fungi! Any one of these creatures could get into the food you prepare on that counter and cause problems.

Be aware that nothing that touches the floor should be allowed to contaminate your countertops.

17.   Drink little or no alcohol.

I know the studies seem conflicting. First it's "Alcohol is bad for you." Then it's "Alcohol is good for you." Who are you to believe?

I've got the answer. Believe as much of the science that is credible that you can. Here are the REAL alcohol facts:

Alcohol Facts

Alcohol consumption is associated with breast and colon cancer.

Alcohol may save you from hepatitis A in raw fish if you drink the alcohol before or while you eat the fish.

Alcohol is a poison and your liver desperately tries to detoxify it.

Alcohol is absorbed in your stomach.

Women have less alcohol dehydrogenase
(an important enzyme in alcohol breakdown) and therefore get drunk faster or more easily.

You can build up a tolerance to a small amount of alcohol.

Even small amounts of alcohol can cause serious birth defects.

Red wine has *Resveratrol*, a potent antioxidant compound that helps keep your cholesterol levels down (you can also get this compound from grape juice).

On balance, I think there is compelling evidence to drink in moderation or not at all. An occasional glass of wine won't hurt you (unless you're pregnant), and may do some good in limited circumstances. Other than that, I avoid alcohol altogether.

18.   Avoid microbes!

Door knobs, public restrooms, handshakes, kisses, dining out, or even eating at home - all could be the source of that one deadly microbe that does you in. My advice for avoiding microbes is as follows.

Wash Often! - Carry antiseptic towelettes with you and use them regularly throughout the day. This is especially important before eating.

Touch nothing! - Open doors and push buttons with knuckles, gloved hands, elbows, feet - anything but fingertips.

Clean/cook food well! - Wash all food well, and make certain all of your food is cooked well before eating it.

Purchase good-looking food. - Select attractive-looking whole foods. Don't look for cheap meat or produce.

Restrooms - Try not to get your hands dirty in public restrooms. More importantly, avoid other people's germs as much as possible. Remember that faucets and doorknobs are covered with bacteria and viruses!

Avoid sick people. - I'm not trying to be cruel, just maintain as much distance as possible. Droplet nuclei are fine droplets of body fluids released into the air when we breathe, cough, or sneeze. Loaded with contagion, they can remain suspended in the air for hours, even days. Gravitate away from coughs and sneezes to avoid breathing the droplet nuclei. Mints may also help, as they have antimicrobial properties.

Food establishments - Watch deli clerks, butchers, chefs, servers, or any other person handling food; their hands should never touch above the neckline (i.e., nose, eyes, mouth, etc.). If you can't see into the kitchen, the surroundings should give you an idea of management's idea of cleanliness. Don't eat in a dirty place!

Food selection - In the supermarket, avoid dented cans, grey/green/purple meat, old food, or any food whose container or box is open. These are all indications of (or invitations for) bacterial contamination.

19.   Laugh loud and often.

It is said that several hours of hearty laughter are equivalent to the 15 minutes of aerobics that you should be doing each day. I recommend laughter, not as a substitute for your exercise, but as a supplement to exercise. If you have no sense of humor, GET ONE!! You're killing yourself without laughter!! There must be something you find funny.

I must say, though, that I have met several people in my lifetime who have absolutely no sense of humor. Is it genetic, forced, environmental? I don't know, but I will say this: most of them are or have been seriously ill. A connection? I think so. Hearty laughter is a complete release of emotion, and necessary for health.

20.   Love someone or some wonderful creature.

Without love, what have you got? **I don't mean the getting of love, but the giving of love!** It doesn't have to be for the perfect mate; it can be love for a neighbor, a friend, a grandmother or a pet. The world needs your help! You can make the world a better place by being a friend to someone or some wonderful creature. See how kind you can be, how much of yourself you can share. I guarantee your emotional life, and subsequently your immune system, will improve.

21.   Get married or live with someone.

Marriage saves countless men from the ravages of disease, according to several credible studies. It appears to do a little less in that department for women, though. Women get health benefits from marriage, if fewer. I think the reason that they do not get as much out of it as men do is because they have to do much of the emotional nurturing, and get less emotional nurturing in return. This whole thing is explained fairly well in John Gray's Men Are From Mars, Women Are From Venus. It is still so important to have someone special that cares about you or you care about, LIVING WITH YOU.

Just live with someone. It can be a friend, sibling, parent, lover, child, or some combination. But the presence of other human beings raises the chances of your being exempt from the ravages of disease. Try not to live alone, far away from people. Get to know your neighbors. We're all in this together.

22.   Avoid radiation.

From the controversial EMF to diagnostic x-rays, try to keep your lifetime radiation exposure as low as possible. As we discuss in Chapter 20, you are allowed up to 10 Rads of radiation in a lifetime before it kills you. This is a little daunting, since radiation is not detectable by the human senses. There are, however several common-sense ways to minimize exposures.

Don't sleep next to electrical appliances or sit too close to the TV. Don't live next to power lines or substations. Minimize contact with radioisotopes if working in the radiological, biological or environmental fields, and measure and keep tabs on your exposure levels. Have your home tested for radon, and install a mitigation system if levels are high.

One of our largest elective radiation exposures is for x-rays. There are numerous cases of individuals getting excessive doses of radiation from improper use of x-ray machines. For example, a four-view mammogram requires an exposure of 0.18 rads. Ask your x-ray technicians what the planned dose is. If they can't tell you, go someplace else.

23.   Seek out and surround yourself with happy people.

The old adage, "Misery loves company" is very true. Misery is a very powerful emotion, and a miserable person (you know the type: a whiner; someone who's always having some sort of devastating crisis; someone always depressed) will only drag you down with them.

Several years ago, I hesitantly brought my very first book to a "friend" of our family who was very interested in the particular subject, and all she said after skimming it and looking at the cover was, "Who's gonna want that?!" After I went home and had a good cry, I decided to find out exactly who would want that, in defiance of her dire prediction. Many thousands of copies and a new career later, I realized that avoiding miserable people was absolutely necessary in my life.

This does not mean you should run when anyone you know has a personal tragedy; on the contrary, you should seek to help other people in order to find personal happiness. It merely means that you should select your constant companions carefully. It will affect your health.

In order to put you in a frame of mind to lay out your life carefully to set up positive attitudes, you need to find the nicest, happiest person you can and try and pattern after them. Don't stalk them, just watch and learn how you could make your personal interactions healthier and happier.

Don't know anyone like that, but still want to try? I've got an even better alternative: Tony Robbins. Tony is one of the best motivational advisors I know. If you really want to change your life for the better, but are unsure how to get started, buy one of his paperbacks. At a cost of about $15 for one of his books in the bookstore or about $180 for his Personal Power II system, it couldn't be more worth your money!

24.   Get 8 hours of sleep a night.

Sleep allows your body to heal and to prepare for the activity of the next day. A very cruel cat experiment that shows the necessity of sleep was performed several years ago. Cats were taken and

deprived of REM (Rapid Eye Movement) sleep. REM sleep is the
sleep time during which we dream. All of the cats who were
wakened continually after they fell asleep, before they got to the
REM cycle, died within days of the experiments. This REM cycle
in humans usually requires at least 4 to 5 hours to reach, that's why
8 hours is recommended.

25.   Exercise!

Want to raise your HDL cholesterol, lower your LDL? Exercise!
Want to have better moods, better sex, a better life in general?
Exercise! Want to slow the aging process dramatically? Want to
live a long and healthy life? I think you know what the answer is;
Exercise!

Chapter 19
VEGETARIANISM

This chapter is particularly geared toward individuals considering vegetarianism, and secondarily for current vegetarians concerned about meeting their nutritional needs. Vegetarianism is a practice you can begin gradually, phasing out meat as you find acceptable nutrient replacements.

Why Go Vegetarian?

People practice vegetarianism for different reasons.

For Health
Vegetarianism is currently thought to provide one with the healthiest fare in terms of cancer and disease prevention. We know that certain aspects of a vegetarian diet make it much more desirable than one that includes the dead flesh of other creatures. Some individuals are concerned about the large amount of drugs and antibiotics given animals that we eat.

For Emotional Reasons
Some vegetarians believe that the killing of animals is barbaric and an atavistic throwback to the times when humans weren't clever enough to cultivate and grow their own crops.. Some find conditions and methods of slaughter so cruel that they do not wish to have any complicity in such acts.

For Environmental Reasons

Some feel that raising animals wastes millions of acres of productive land and the clearing of such land destroys the habitats of the earth. Still others realize that to get the most protein from the earth, plants are the only way to go because it takes 21 pounds of plant protein to make one pound of muscle (meat protein) in a cow. The ratio is a bit lower for smaller animals, but so much fertile land is wasted that it needs consideration.

For Religious Reasons

Then there are those whose religious beliefs do not permit the consumption of dead animal flesh, such as the Seventh Day Adventists and Hindus.

Types of Vegetarians

There has been a lot of discussion about vegetarian diets lately and there are a lot of misconceptions. First, there are four types of vegetarians:

Vegans - The strictest type of vegetarian, a vegan will only consume foods that contain no animal products or byproducts. This requires careful planning and the reading of labels of all foods, as many "meatless" foods contain meat stock, meat-derived fats, or dairy products. This diet requires much discipline.

Fruitarians - They eat only fruits, honey, nuts and oils. This group represents a relatively small percentage of vegetarians. A true fruitarian diet is potentially dangerous because of lack of protein and other nutrient issues.

Lactovegetarians - This type of vegetarian eats only vegetables, fruits and dairy products. This is a modification of the vegan diet that allows the addition of cheese and milk as protein sources.

Ovolactovegetarians - This type of vegetarian eats vegetables, fruits, dairy products like cheese, and eggs (and pasta!). The addition of eggs opens up a whole world of proteinaceous foods left out of the other types of vegetarian diets. It is relatively easy to be an ovolactovegetarian and have a very full diet.

Benefits of a Vegetarian Diet

Vegetarians potentially reap enormous benefits in terms of reduced rates of heart disease and cancer, as well as overall well-being. Plant foods are, for the most part, low in calories, lower in protein, and can even be low in fats.

Plant foods also have NO CHOLESTEROL!! They <u>never have had</u> any cholesterol, because it is a strictly animal compound. But, as we mentioned elsewhere, cholesterol is not the main culprit when your cholesterol reading is high. The bad guys are (too much) saturated fat or (too much) fat in general in your diet. I always advise my students and clients to forget about cholesterol in their foods and watch for overall fat content. Shoot for lowering your fat to about 30 grams per day.

There's nothing to eat but spaghetti!

I have had this statement made countless times in my Nutrition classes, and it couldn't be farther from the truth! I will list here just a few of the possibilities. There are virtually limitless food choices in a vegetarian diet! Enough to satisfy even the most voracious meat eater. You can substitute egg, cheese, tofu, chick peas, other vegetables or TVP (textured vegetable protein) when you feel that a meat substitute is needed.

Experimenting is the key to successful vegetarianism!

Foods You Can Eat On An Ovolactovegetarian Diet
(* - Vegetarian substitutes for meat items)

American/Italian classics

All breads,rolls, etc.
Hamburgers*
Omelettes
Spaghetti
Grilled cheese
Barbequed foods
Fettucini

Sausages*
Lasagna
Pizza
Peanut butter
Mashed potatoes
Linguine

Chinese classics

Chow Mein
Egg Drop Soup
Sweet and Sour Vegetables
Broccoli with garlic sauce
Boiled rice
Sauteed bamboo shoots and mushrooms

Moo Shu
Wonton Soup
Cashew vegetables
Vegetable fried rice
Tea

Japanese classics

Maki sushi
California roll
Tempura
Soba Tsuyu

Bara sushi
Teriyaki vegetables
Rice

Indian classics

Pakoras
Papadum
Korma
Naan
Sabzi pilau

Mulligatawney soup
Raita
Tandoori specialties
Onion paneer kulcha
Gaajar Aur Sooay Ki Bhaji

The foods above are just a few of the possibilities you should explore for yourself. Ask your grocer to carry them if you can't find them! Indian food, in particular, has a rich history of vegetarian cuisine. Any dish can be made vegetarian, although some dishes convert more successfully and some cooks are more successful at the conversion.

Possible Deficiencies in the Vegetarian Diet

Let's be frank, all diets have some deficiencies. That's why I sometimes recommend a multivitamin/mineral supplement every three days or so. No type of diet is perfect, but the minute you begin restricting any sort of food from your intake, that's when you need to be careful. Below are some of the possible deficiencies that a vegetarian who's not careful might have.

Possible Vegetarian Deficiencies

Vitamins
Riboflavin
Vitamin B-12
Vitamin D

Minerals
Zinc
Iron
Calcium

Energy-Yielding Nutrients
Protein

To overcome these deficiencies, vegetarians can use a vegetarian multiple vitamin or specific vitamin or mineral supplement that complements their diet.

Vitamins deficient in the Vegetarian Diet
A **Vitamin D** deficiency can be overcome by allowing 15 minutes per day in full sunlight because we can manufacture our own Vitamin D through sunlight on our skin.

Riboflavin and **Vitamin B-12** deficiencies can be overcome with foods and supplementation. But what can appear to be a B-12 deficiency can be a result of **Folate** deficits. The B vitamins are often hard to separate from one another as far as deficiencies go.

We need 2 - 3 micrograms of Vitamin B-12 per day. Vitamin B-12 can be found in milk (about 1 microgram per serving), eggs (3 -10 micrograms per serving), fermented cheese (1 - 3 micrograms per serving), and pickles (0.5 micrograms per serving). Vitamin B-12 is also manufactured by bacteria in a healthy intestine. Eating yogurt will go a long way to keeping intestinal flora intact. Riboflavin can be found in milk, enriched breakfast cereals and breads, and mushrooms.

Minerals deficient in the Vegetarian Diet
Zinc deficiency can be avoided by eating extra nutmeats in the diet or supplementation with chewable zinc gluconate or zinc sulfate tablets. **Iron** deficiency is found in omnivorous diets as well as vegetarian ones. Blackstrap molasses, raisins, green peas and any fortified bread or rice (most of our bread and rice is fortified) can solve the deficiency. Again, occasional supplementation is not unheard of. But it should not be long-term unless you suffer from serious anemia or another serious disease which requires it.

One of the issues in the vegetarian diet is one which involves insoluble fiber and phytates (mentioned in the Carbohydrate chapter). It is the issue of minerals lost due to binding with these carbohydrates. **Calcium** is one of those easily bonded minerals. To avoid calcium deficiency, vegetarians should eat their yogurt (or calcium-laden foods like almonds) separate from large quantities of fiber. At a different time of day, for example. That's one of the reasons that "Raisin bran with 100% of your vitamins" is false advertising. You cannot absorb or even hold onto those vitamins when they are taken along with bran. It's a nice, but empty gesture.

Protein Deficiency in the Vegetarian Diet
Vegetarians always wear this invisible sign around their neck that only carnivores see. It says, "I'm not getting enough protein, can you help me? Maybe I should eat some meat?" A careful vegetarian knows the limiting amino acids, mostly lysine and methionine, and uses combinations such as rice and beans to get complete protein. It is not difficult with practice. Vegetarians often gesture at the most muscled of all the animals in the kingdom, the elephant. He eats only leaves and grasses yet has plenty of protein to build and sustain his large muscles. So protein deficiency is not as big an issue as once thought.

"Vegetarians always seem so thin and unhealthy." This is a myth perpetuated by those who favor beefy diets. We all know that big isn't necessarily better anyway. Can you get fat on a vegetarian diet? Absolutely! Any time you eat more than you burn off, storage as fat occurs. If you eat a lot of food, you should also beware of the avocado and other fruits like it that are very high in saturated fat. Certain other plants and nuts are high in fat and nutritious components as well. This is good news for the vegetarian who eats moderately and bad news for those who eat too much.

Vegans often tend to have a lifestyle that is compatible with long, healthy living. This often includes exercise, non-smoking, and no caffeine or alcohol. Enough cannot be said about the way we live.

Every choice you make either comes back to haunt you or helps you on your goal to good health.

What is good health? Well, the old definition that is still tossed around is "the absence of active disease". This definition just doesn't cut it anymore. We all know that exercise is unavoidable for good health. Good health, to me, is the presence of vigor and ability to tolerate moderate exercise, along with the absence of visible or non-visible disease. "I haven't been to see the doctor in months; I never get colds anymore;"... None of these are signs of good health as defined here. If you want good health, eat vegetarian and exercise!

Vegetarianism
To Wage War

1) Buy only vegetarian foods.
2) Tell the store and restaurant managers that you need more vegetarian choices.
3) Hold vegetarian events at local malls, health food stores, restaurants, etc.
5) If your reasons for being vegetarian are moral, join organizations like PETA, etc. for vegetarian support.
6) Subscribe to Vegetarian Times (800-829-3340).

TORPEDOES

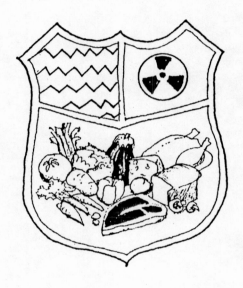

Chapter 20
FOOD IRRADIATION

Now that we've talked about microbes in your food, you may have heard that the answer to all our troubles is to irradiate everything. Well, guess again. This is just the dangerous knee-jerk over-reaction of those in the food industry. They are reacting out of fear that someone in this increasing litigious society will sue them for illness or death resulting from consumption of their product. And, in a way you can't blame them. I'm sure if your small child died from eating lunch at a fast-food restaurant, you'd be pretty distraught. But lawsuits and irradiation are not the answer. Good Manufacturing Practices (GMP) are.

If Good Manufacturing Practices (rules commonly used in industry to set reasonable standards with which to properly create food products) were to include all of the practices outlined in the Food Safety chapter, you might never have to worry about microbes in your food again. These suggestions are just too difficult for the food industry to swallow, economically speaking. Irradiation is just cheaper, plain and simple. And cheap is the way most manufacturers want to go. The prevailing wisdom is, "To hell with the future, this works now and will save us transition time, education, and legal fees."

But food manufacturers are trading your future health for their present comfort. Irradiation is known to cause cancer, just like cigarettes are. Ultraviolet and x-ray irradiation are two good examples of radiation that we know causes us cancer. We know very little about the radiation coming off our food. To be fair, there is always some small amount of background radiation present in our environment. I am not making reference to this small amount of radiation; I am talking about something that exists *after* background radiation is subtracted.

How Does Irradiation Work?

Food products are bombarded with gamma rays from radioactive isotopes like Cobalt-60. These isotopes most often come from nuclear waste. Since nuclear waste is so profoundly mutagenic and cancer-causing, food scientists thought, "Hey, I'll bet this stuff would kill bacteria!", and "Eureka!" a bad idea was born. Irradiation does kill bacteria and some viruses in our food supply. That's good. But it's also bad because its mutagenic power could also be our undoing.   Irradiation could help replace several pesticides and anti-fungal compounds used on our produce. But so could careful harvesting and extra cleanliness.

There are several irradiation plants in the U.S. As of 1992, 40 countries (including the U.S.) allowed irradiation. According to Rosanna Morrison in the December 1992 issue of the USDA Food Review, complacency about microorganisms may result once the food has been sterilized. There is no lasting anti-microbial benefit to irradiation. Even the rays given off by the irradiated food do not kill most microorganisms.   Sterilized food may even be more susceptible to takeover by food illness organisms because the indigenous microorganisms that might compete for resources have been removed.

And much of the contamination in your meats and cheeses is a result of the deli-clerk or the butcher standing right in front of you at the supermarket. **This contamination happens AFTER irradiated food is sent to the stores.** I once witnessed a deli-clerk come around from behind the counter to greet a friend of hers who was a new mother. The mother said she had to run and get something and asked if the clerk would watch the baby. So she did. But the baby had an accident and the clerk was forced to clean up the diarrhea and rediaper the baby. I watched her closely as she wiped some of the diarrhea off her hands with a cloth towel from the diaper bag. The mother returned and the clerk went back behind the counter and offered to get me any cold cuts I wanted. I declined, not knowing what to say as the next woman in line ordered her half pound of ham. Irradiation won't solve this issue.

Years later, as a Board of Health inspector (traveling incognito), I asked a veteran butcher in a grocery store why he was not wearing gloves to cut the meat. His reply, "I can't get the feel of the meat with gloves on. Those health people don't know what they're talking about. This meat is fine. Gloves won't help. Besides when no one's looking we all just take them off anyway." This is the front line. Irradiation will not help you from getting sick from Salmonella or Hepatitis from the filthy hands of a butcher or deli-clerk who has poor personal hygiene. Only education and enforcement can solve that problem.

In a recent paper in <u>Trends in Food Science and Technology</u> (Vol. 3, 1992), M. H. Stevenson of the Food and Agricultural Chemistry Research Division in Northern Ireland elucidated the methods by which radiation can be detected from foods that have been irradiated. The three methods of detecting radiation coming off your food are **thermoluminescence, electron spin resonance spectroscopy** (ESR), and **chemical analysis** of the formation of long chain hydrocarbons from lipids in the food.

<u>**Thermoluminescence**</u> is the phenomenon whereby food that has been irradiated gives off a low level of light. This light is the conversion of electron energy into what is known as a photon, or particle of light. Photons are not normally given off from your

food. The detection of this light allows one to determine if a given food has been irradiated or not.

Herbs and spices are irradiated twice to determine if the source is soil deposits or the plants themselves. Surprised? I didn't realize, either, that all of our spices are now (and have been) irradiated for years without our knowledge or permission... "For our safety..."

Electron Spin Resonance (ESR) Spectroscopy is used because "When food is treated with ionizing radiation, free radicals are formed." (Stevenson, 1992). *Free Radicals* are pro-oxidants, the agents we fight against all of our lives with antioxidants and nutrition. They are the chemical agents of CANCER! O.K., so now we know they're found in your food. What foods? Fruits, meat, shellfish, spices, and as many foods as the governments will allow. The free radicals can be measured after irradiation, according to this paper.

IRRADIATED FOOD MAY IRRADIATE YOU!!

That's what some of you will take home from this discussion!! It may be an overreaction or it may end up being right on the money. After all, photons, free radicals, active and unusual lipid compounds are present in your irradiated foods. In order for food safety inspectors to test if a food like chicken or spices has been irradiated, they must measure it with a device that measures these changes. That's right, your chicken gives off photons in the freezer case, in your cart, and in your bags on the way home. It doesn't stop there. The radiation it gives off can be measured after you clean it, cook it, AND SERVE AND EAT IT!!! In other words the particles that result from the killing and mutation of the surface bacteria and the entire food are now pressing themselves onto your mouth, esophagus, and intestinal tissue as you ingest the food. Who knows what sort of cancer you might be able to look forward to if you eat the right amount of irradiated food?

Chemical Analysis of Lipids involves looking for those unusual compounds that are formed upon irradiation. According to Stevenson, "Irradiation can induce a number of chemical changes in the fatty acids found in foods." **New compounds are formed.** These compounds include hydrocarbons with one additional double bond more than the parent compound, or one or two carbons less. The main compounds used as markers are **tetradecene, hexacadecadiene, 2-alkylcyclobutanones,** and **heptadecene.** The amounts of these increase with increasing doses of radiation. Alkylcyclobutanones such as **2-dodecylcyclobutanone** (which arises from palmitic acid) and **2-tetradecylcyclobutanone** (from stearic acid) have been found in chicken meat as a result of irradiation.

The alkylcyclobutanones are known agents with cancer-causing potential. And now they will be in your chicken, beef, pork and eggs. **And all you had to do to kill all the bacteria in your food was cook it properly!!!** But the government is afraid of lawsuits. It is easier to tell you "You will never be able to learn how to properly cook your food; we must irradiate it for you."

Does It Affect Your DNA?

Possibly. All living creatures have DNA inside each cell of each organ. There is DNA in your wheat cereal, your hamburger, your banana. When we consume DNA from foods, it is mostly broken down into harmless components - or is it? Straight DNA, outside of the organism in which it was made, has mechanisms in place in order to be reabsorbed into living creatures. This is especially true of the transfer of DNA or RNA from bacterium-to-bacterium and viruses-into-anything. When we speak of the possible transmission of viruses from your food to you, we are talking about the transfer of DNA or RNA to your cells. When you get a cold or the flu, DNA or RNA from some rhinovirus or adenovirus has penetrated your eye, nose or mouth epithelial cells and has tried to tell them what to do. You fight back with lots of mucus and sneezing to get rid of the little buggers, but in the end, your immune system must take charge for you to be healthy again.

DNA analysis of your food reveals irradiation and freeze-thawing changes as well. The DNA in the cells of the chicken you are about to eat may be changed enough by radiation to make it dangerous to you. Odd proteins could be formed. This unusual DNA made by irradiation could incorporate itself into your cells. There is, however, a type of DNA in all cells (our cells _and_ chicken cells) that generally resists breakdown and cannot be changed by these assaults. It is your mitochondrial DNA. Found in an organelle that we only get from our mothers, it alone is protected. Thanks, mom.

Does It Produce Free Radicals?

Yes. In "Irradiated Foods", a bulletin from the American Council On Science and Health (1996), it is stated that the ionizing radiation used on food produces **ions**, **free radicals**, and **excited molecules**. These are chemically active compounds that can produce other changes in a product besides the killing of bacteria - changes that might be harmful over time or toxic in the short term.

Does It Affect The Nutritional Value Of The Food?

Yes. It has been found that high doses of radiation cause **vitamin loss** as well as changes in lipid content and protein molecules.

But the most serious question to ask is whether it actually works.

Does It Work? Does It Sterilize Your Food To A Safe Level?

In the bulletin described above, it is suggested that **the risk of food poisoning might actually increase** because typical spoilage organisms that produce odors we recognize would be killed, while other pathogenic organisms might survive. **So it looks OK, smells OK, but is contaminated with serious pathogens?** That leaves you with NO warning, just having to trust what the government tells you. Not a good idea.

What Are The Concentrations Of Radiation In Your Life?

A RAD is a measure of the ionizing radiation absorbed by your tissues. We are exposed to a certain amount of radiation in various forms as a "background" dose. These forms include cosmic rays from space, and radon from the decay of radionuclides in the soil or rock. **Your Maximum Lifetime exposure should be limited to 10 RADS, if possible.**

1 kGy =	100,000 RAD =	1/10 of a megaRAD
10 kGy =	1,000,000 RAD =	1 megaRAD
1 RAD =	1000milliRAD =	1/1,000,000 of a megaRAD
10 RAD =	10,000milliRAD =	1/100,000 of a megaRAD

Your yearly background dose	350-500milliRAD
An airplane ride	1-5 milliRAD / Hour
A Mammogram	180-300milliRAD
A chest X-ray	40 milliRAD
A Thyroid scan*	200 RAD
very localized	

Irradiation Doses Used on Foods (USDA Food Review 1992)
The units of irradiation used are called Kilograys (kGy).

0.05 - 0.15 kGy	Potatoes, asparagus
0.30 - 0.75 kGy	For insect infestation
0.10 - 0.75 kGy	To delay fruit ripening
1.0 - 2.0 kGy	For microbes in fish, fungi in fruit
1.5 - 3.0 kGy	For microbes in meat and poultry
10.0 - 30.0 kGy	For microbes in spices
23.0 - 57.0 kGy	For unrefrigerated storage

10 kGy is considered, by proponents of irradiation, to be the limit of safety. Notice the amount used on spices and unrefrigerated foods.

Irradiation
To Wage War

1) Insist on labelling on all foods that are irradiated.
2) Insist on an adequate explanation of all of the dangers of food irradiation from the USDA and FDA.
3) Oppose any plans for the irradiation of new foods until you are assured of their safety.
4) Contact the companies in your area that irradiate foods; they should be fairly easy to find. Get their literature and read it carefully. If there is anything that makes no sense, discuss it with a local consumer reporter.
5) Talk to anyone and everyone who will listen.
6) Organize a consumer group that gets answers to these questions.
7) Buy spices from companies that do not irradiate like The Spice Hunter, Inc. San Luis Obispo, California (800) 444-3061.
8) Do not buy or consume irradiated foods.

Chapter 21
BIOTECHNOLOGY

What is genetically engineered food?
Genetically engineered food is a vegetable crop (e.g., carrots) or animal (e.g., pigs) which has had its DNA altered in order to produce more of a certain product (e.g., beta-carotene) or enhance a certain quality that will make the average shopper purchase more. The almighty dollar is mostly what motivates such food changes.

Initially, genetic engineering was thought to be a good thing, creating pest-resistant crops, larger produce, longer-lasting foods. Not anymore. It is a messy nightmare of foreign insects and plants released into areas with no place in the ecosystem, the willy-nilly spraying of bacterial slurries all over our crops at a time when Vice President Al Gore says he is trying to get rid of bacterial illnesses in the U.S. food supply, and unusual creations. These unusual creations include proteins which are antigenic (induce an immune system alert!) or toxic.

Allergens can cause serious problems, according to an article in the May 1996 New England Journal of Medicine. And as Marian Burros, a New York Times reporter, said in a May 1997 article, "For those with unusual allergies,... there is no way to know what foods to avoid." From the same New York Times article:

"Genetic engineers are taking genes from bacteria, viruses and insects and adding them to fruits, grains and vegetables," said Dr. Rebecca Goldburg, an Environmental Defense Fund senior scientist. "They are producing foods that have never before been eaten by human beings. Consumers should not be guinea pigs for untested food substances." (Burros, 1997)

Pig genes in my broccoli?
Other unusual creations to which I strongly object are <u>transgenic</u> organisms. Transgenic organisms have genes from some other member of the animal kingdom inserted into their DNA. Mostly we find researchers inserting animal genes into produce. This is cause for concern. We don't know what effect these transfers from animal to vegetable will have on our safety.

If a vegetarian, for example, is bound by religion or creed to never eat meat, has he/she violated that oath as a result of the consumption of a carrot? And how is he/she supposed to know that there are pig genes and pig products in his/her potato or broccoli? There is no way to know unless such products are prohibited in the market or carefully labeled.

An advertisement for a Transgenic Nutraceuticals conference came to me in the mail the other day. I was appalled. It's not as if some careful planning went into this idea. The food scientists just want to monkey around some more to improve the profits in the industry. Even those at the pinnacle of this transgenic research will admit that we don't know everything that might happen as a result of our overwhelming desire to sell products. And I'm sure some of those transgenic nutraceuticals would fall under the heading of Antioxidant Secret #1, and instead create disease situations similar to those they might have prevented had plants and pigs been left to their own devices.

Those who advocate the genetic engineering of food always call out the name of Gregor Mendel in order to cloak themselves in sound scientific precedent. Not so fast, fellas. We all know that Mendel was the first real geneticist, combining pollen from one type of pea plant with another to create a new strain. We also know he did this many times until he was satisfied with both the result and the simplistic understanding of how it came about. He was, in effect, aiding nature. Farmers had done this for years even before Mendel came close to figuring out how it works. But he could never have imagined such a rapidly changing revolution in both crop and farm animal production. And I'm sure his curiosity would have been preceded by caution when approaching such a vast unknown area.

Foods That Are Genetically Engineered Today**

** According to "Eating Well" by Marian Burros, (NYTimes, May 1997) whose source was Genetic ID of Fairfield, Iowa, these are foods that were found to be positive for genetically engineered ingredients. These were the only foods tested; there are many more foods that may be genetically engineered. Contact Genetic ID if you want to learn about specific foods. The FDA has said it feels such foods are safe.

Soybeans (13-16% of our supply*)
Soy Foods
Carnation™ Alsoy Baby Formula
Similac™ Neocare Baby Formula
Isomil™ Baby Formula
Enfamil™ Prosbee Baby Formula
Morningstar Farms™ Breakfast Links
Morningstar Farms™ Better'n Burgers
Betty Crocker™ Bacos Bacon Bits

Corn (2% of all U.S. supply*)
Corn Foods
Fritos™
Tostitos™ Crispy Rounds
Doritos™ Nacho Cheesier Chips

Is it improving our food supply?
I recently took my nine-year old neighbor, Jessica, to the supermarket and showed her the produce section. "What's this?" I

asked her as I held the fruit up. "A strawberry" she expectedly
replied. "No, I wish it were a strawberry. A strawberry is a
conical fruit, small and tasty. This is a big lumpy, pasty, nearly
tasteless excuse for a strawberry. It looks red enough and provides
the farmer with extra cash cause it's so big, but that's about all it
has to offer", I replied. "I'm going to show you a real strawberry
later." She knows I'm always on a mission and finds the whole
thing amusing. Later I gave her one of the berries from my wild
patch in the back yard. "Wow. That's tasty!" she said.

Strawberries have been genetically engineered for years. The
result is poor-tasting, but big berries. I also wonder if the
antioxidants found in non-engineered strawberries aren't destroyed
with all of this manipulation. And so does someone else
apparently; a September 1997 bulletin in the Bloomberg News
announced the discovery that wild blueberries contain much higher
concentrations of antioxidants than cultivated ones. Be aware that
following this report some food scientist will attempt to engineer
the berries' DNA to change all that! I wonder, then, if farmers
grow strawberries to have more Vitamin C, will the berries have a
toxic protein only discovered after some hapless consumer serves
them for dinner?

The National PTA (Parent-Teacher Association) voted in March of
1995 to allow milk tainted with the addition of recombinant BST
(a milk production hormone) to be given to school children. Under
pressure from one of the strongest lobbyists in the food industry
(the Institute of Food Technologists) and in an effort to show that
they were not afraid of new technology, they caved in to one of the
worst ideas the food industry has come up with yet. This
genetically engineered hormone will be used to cause cows to
produce twice as much milk as normal. It's not bad enough that
there is too much milk produced in this country, and our taxes pay
for much of it to be dumped, but our children will be consuming

this genetically engineered milk! It is also very taxing on the cows who are not made to hold that much milk in their udders. It is a disgrace.

Is it dangerous?
We put our faith in genetic engineering every time we eat yogurt or cheese because the bacteria used to produce the products is altered continually with a foreign piece of DNA called a plasmid. Because this inserted piece of DNA is foreign to the bacteria, the bacteria tries to "shed" or get rid of it, so new ones have to be created and inserted. We hope there are no mistakes, but occasionally things do happen.

Renegade proteins that can cause severe allergic reactions, toxic proteins that might severely harm susceptible individuals, and lots of other possibilities exist in this unknown realm. "Hey, the scientists know what they're doing..." Oh, yeah? I'm a scientist and have seen the sloppy research that goes on in food science. I have seen how ignorant we really are about what to do inside a cell nucleus. Molecular biologists with advanced degrees have a fairly comprehensive knowledge about DNA manipulation, but the average food scientist does not! And they're all getting into it now! Sure they have restriction endonucleases, micromanipulative tools, electrophoretic gels. But do they really know what they might create if they insert a nucleotide sequence improperly?

Science is serendipity. That is an important concept. But it must also try and restrict itself to necessary, careful research that does not involve an unwitting public. Food scientists should not be doing molecular experiments they do not fully comprehend! I attended one meeting about the subject and was appalled at the lack of basic knowledge about molecular issues.

Is biotechnology dangerous? Ask the Swiss government. The Swiss had to recall Toblerone™ bars recently because they were made with genetically engineered soybeans and the result was an unnatural compound that made antibiotics less effective. Could other genetically engineered foods produce these effects? Who knows? It should be enough to breed and test the effects of traits without getting into the nucleus of each organism.

Genetic engineering is not always a bad thing, though. It has brought us many important products like insulin for diabetics. It is a useful scientific advance, if properly monitored. For a long time scientists just bombarded food with mutagenic substances and then took the one from a group of hundreds that had the desired characteristics. "Spray and pray" is the industry term for this willy nilly bombardment. Lately there are more specific techniques using target genes and inserted DNA. Not safer, just more specific.

Biotechnology
To Wage War

1)   Insist on labelling of food that has been genetically engineered.

2)   Use your purchasing power to send a message.

3)   Call the companies who make your favorite foods.

Chapter 22
PESTICIDES

Pesticide History

Early pesticides were the cornerstone of crop management for hundreds of years. These "first generation" pesticides were used all over the world to eliminate pest problems. Many were ineffective; others proved to be extremely toxic. Ground tobacco, sulfur and ash were commonly used.

Arsenic was used in China at the turn-of-the-century to control locust invasions; it is still used surreptitiously in third world countries to control insect populations. And you may be sitting on one of the largest sources of arsenic that consumers are exposed to, your picnic table, benches, and the deck attached to your house. These are soaked with an arsenic spray to prevent decay and insect infestation. Still think it isn't a food problem for you? Well, if you ever eat fish, there is a very good chance that arsenic will show up in your blood, presumably partly because other countries are using and dumping arsenic compounds in that largest, most abused of dumping grounds, the ocean.

The dawn of a new era of pest management was upon us with the creation of pesticides in the lab via organic synthesis. Just ask Rachel Carson readers (and read her book, Silent Spring). These chemicals initially appeared to be non-toxic; DDT was even used to dust and delouse soldiers in World War II.

FEDERAL FOOD REGULATIONS

Federal Food, Drug, and Cosmetic Act (FFDCA, Section 408)
Federal Insecticide, Fungicide, and Rodenticide Act (FIFRA)
If a pesticide is registered under FIFRA, the FFDCA / EPA allows
tolerance limits of the pesticide that fit the usage in the registration. Nice.
Hey, that's not the fox guarding the henhouse, is it?   As a
pharmaceutical/pesticide producer, all you have to do to cover the large
amounts of pesticide in the ultimate product is to list a "necessary"
pesticide concentration much greater than you'd ever expect farmers to
use on crops. This is for processed food.

FFDCA (Section 409)
A pesticide is considered a "food additive" under this section used for raw
foods. This section applies to preservatives, sweeteners, and the raw
produce in fruit juices, flours, tomato paste and other raw food
commodities.   Sections 408 and 409 are linked by a "flow-through"
provision which allows residues of pesticides to be considered O.K. if the
manufacturer promises to remove as much pesticide as it can during
processing, or if the pesticide level in the processed food is equal to or
lower than residues registered for in Section 408. This is all that we have
to protect us!   The National Food Processors Association (NFPA) is
regularly up in arms, attempting to undermine the EPA regulations for
safety, stating that there is little proof that pesticides are harmful.

THE DELANEY CLAUSE (Les Vs. Reilly, 1992)
EPA may not allow any level of pesticide in processed food that is greater
than the level found in the same raw food if the pesticide presents any
carcinogenic risk. The basis for argument about allowing new pesticides
is whether the new pesticides will concentrate in processed food, and
whether they fall under this clause.
EPA Journal, March 1993

The Delaney Paradox

I. Are Foods Allowed To Give Us Cancer?

No food additive is allowed that causes cancer
BUT
Pesticides in food are allowed to cause cancer

II. Who Minds The Store?

Additives are covered under FDCA
(Food, Drug and Cosmetic Act)

Pesticides are covered under FIFRA
(Federal Insecticide, Fungicide and Rodenticide Act)

Therefore a risk / benefit analysis is done. If the killing benefit is great to the farmer and the risk is fairly low to the consumer as determined by slanted science; then the law says, "To hell with the consumer".

III. Is There Any Protection From Cancer-Causing Pesticides?

If a cancer-causing pesticide is permitted in food, and then it concentrates, it becomes a food additive and is then covered under FDCA rules. If, for example, a pesticide was allowed in tomatoes which were then used mostly for tomato sauce; it might become disallowed.

IV. And The Problems Are?

A)   Carcinogens are permitted under FIFRA.

B)   Carcinogens are seldom permitted under FDCA (but not never).

C)   Carcinogens used as Feed Additives for livestock, such as hormones and drugs are permitted, whether they are found in the food or not.

Today, well over 1500 different chemical ingredients are used in formulating 33,000+ different pesticide-containing products. These include insecticides, herbicides, fungicides, miticides, and rodenticides. These can be broadly grouped into 3 divisions: chlorinated hydrocarbons; organic phosphates; and carbamates.

The Three Basic Divisions Of Pesticides Currently Used

Chlorinated hydrocarbons
Organic phosphates
Carbamates

Chlorinated Hydrocarbons

The chlorinated hydrocarbons are controversial because they are extremely resistant to breakdown in the environment, are passed up the food chain, and are stored in animal fat. Chlorinated hydrocarbons are capable of causing birth defects, nerve damage, and cancer (Chiras, 1988). Many are currently being reconsidered or banned from widespread use in this country. Third world countries have no such ban.

Examples of Chlorinated Hydrocarbons

DDT	Aldrin	Dieldrin
Chlordane	Lindane	Heptachlor
Endrin	Mirex	Toxaphene

Organophosphates

Organic phosphates, like malathion and parathion, are less likely to be passed up the food chain. Many are toxic to humans, though. High doses cause convulsions, paralysis, tremors, coma and death.

Low doses may cause confusion, diarrhea, vomiting, headaches and breathing difficulty.

Carbamates

Carbamates remain in the environment for a few days to two weeks after application. They are widely used as fungicides, insecticides, and herbicides. Sevin™ (Carbaryl) is an example of a widely used carbamate. These pesticides are neurotoxic and capable of causing genetic damage and birth defects.

Pesticides in Conventionally-Grown Foods

In this section I will use the term "conventional" or "conventionally grown" to refer to crops grown with conventional, man-made pesticides. If you think these just "go away" as part of the growing and harvesting process, you may be surprised to learn the following.

Peaches retain the most pesticide, according to a researcher at Rutgers University. He ran an analysis on most commercial produce and reported the results in several papers. And in a recent analysis by the Environmental Working Group, 7 out of 10 samples of peaches tested positive for a variety of pesticides.

Raisins are a big surprise when it comes to pesticides. According to a recent study, 110 pesticides were found in only 16 commercial samples. As my Grandma Alice would say, that's a lot of "gunk you don't need".

Apples are loaded with a real melange of chemical pesticides. They are also often coated with a potentially cancer-causing wax loaded with fungicides. They have so many pesticides that when I asked a local apple farm if they had an idea of what pesticides they used, they became very angry and said, "What do you need to know for? There are dozens; check with the town hall."

Spinach is known to harbor DDT! I was amazed to find this out. It is still used surreptitiously in this country and openly in other countries like Mexico and countries in South America.

Peppers are regularly sprayed with carbamates, which are active neurotoxins up to two weeks after they're sprayed on the fruit. This means that if your farmer's spraying schedule has them sprayed just before they're picked (and it happens more than you know!), you could be in trouble if you buy and eat them inside that two week period.

What is the effect of pesticides in our food?
Those that remain in the food itself have long been suspected of causing cancer. There is no question that farmers and migrant workers and those exposed to the highest levels show increased risk of developing serious problems from the carcinogenic and toxic effects of such pesticides. Many die each year from direct toxic exposure.

There is no escape from the effects of pesticides in produce. We all eat vegetables. Even if we wash them, there are systemic pesticides we can't remove. We only have ourselves to blame, really. We need to have exotic, tropical fruit in the dead of winter and produce from hundreds of miles away. Long trips or long waits for produce are not without peril; fruit and vegetables ripen and rot very quickly without assistance. It's just that we've gone too far with this "assistance". I don't need that waxed (paraffin causes cancer), lumpy, brown-spotted-under-the-skin delicious apple that's 12 to 14 MONTHS(!) old! I'll wait for the next season, thank you. It's not just fruit. Vegetables like zucchini that keep a little longer are sprayed and waxed as well. Doesn't anybody care?

The government touts its Delaney Clause as the grand, protective measure to insure that <u>known</u> cancer-causing pesticides that concentrate when food is processed are not used on certain crops. What about <u>unknown</u> cancer-causing pesticides? There are **many thousands** more pesticides created each year than the government can keep a handle on. These all fall through the cracks. And that means onto the table and into your loved ones mouths. It's appalling. The Delaney clause also does not cover animals - that we eat. They are forced to eat any old pesticided grain they get. If that isn't bad enough, they eat the non-consumable waste from local food processing companies **AND ONE ANOTHER!** That's correct, the animals you consume as beef, pork and chicken in many cases are forced to become cannibals or die. Therefore the concentration of pesticide in the little grain they actually get is vitally important!

Let's say a concentration of 50 parts per million (ppm) of a given pesticide is toxic to humans and there is only the possibility of the cow getting 35 ppm in its tissues through grain sources. Fine, you say. That's OK. But wait, if cow #1 eats several other cows during the year, ten for example, then the concentration of cancer-causing pesticide in the meat made from the cow #1 is 350 ppm! So what you eat could be far above the toxic limit of 50 ppm!

Who really is among those 4000 people that <u>die</u> every year as a direct result of pesticides in the food? Farmers, migrant workers, and people living on or near a farm that regularly sprays the crops with pesticides. The average consumer is not likely to die immediately as a result of pesticide contamination in his/her produce. Rather, the average consumer will have a slow induction of any number of painful cancers that might result from eating too much pesticide-covered produce. And in this era of "five fruits and five vegetables a day!", it is appalling that farmers still favor the old ways.

The bottom line is that you should search for and begin to demand that you be given food choices that are organically grown. This is the only way you might be safe from pesticide contamination.

Organically Grown Versus Conventionally Grown Produce

Consumer demand for fresh produce is at an all time high. The number of consumers reporting increased consumption of fresh vegetables continues to rise annually. This renewed interest manifests itself in an interest in produce quality. Increased public concern over health and safety has led to an increasing interest in the products of alternative farming methods, most notably "organic" and "low-input" growing techniques.

A food is recognized as "organically grown" by several organizations around the country collectively called NOFA (National Organic Farmers Association). For a food to be classified as organic, it must follow "agricultural methods which promote the biological health of the soils, and without the use of synthetic fertilizers, insecticides, herbicides, fungicides, or rodenticides" (according to NOFA-New Jersey).

Let's pause right here to examine that definition. "Synthetic" pesticides are unacceptable. But did you know that naturally derived pesticides are used? That's right, all organic farmers USE PESTICIDES! I was amazed when I found out, but after working in the fields for four years, I understand. Some of these acceptable organic pesticides are quite toxic, though. In fact one that was recently removed from most lists of acceptable organic pesticides-Rotenone-caused all the fish in a lake or stream except carp (who can gulp air at the surface of the water) to suffocate and drown. It suppressed the nervous system excitation of the fishes' gills.

There are a number of facts to keep in mind when considering going organic. David Pimentel of Cornell University explained them quite clearly in a 1990 wide-ranging study of the use and effectiveness of pesticides.

His study showed that 20,000 people a year are poisoned by pesticides. Many of these die. Most are either living near or working with farms or agricultural crops. It is a tragedy that need not occur.

"Agricultural chemicals have become increasingly counter-productive. The tonnage of pesticides applied to U.S. croplands has grown 33-fold since the 1940's" (Briefings, 1991). Crop losses have actually increased to almost 40% during the same period of time. This is due to insect resistance and single-crop farmers. Crop rotation and biological pest control could allow reduction of pesticides by half the current level of usage.

A recent book by Michael W. Fox called "Superpigs and Wondercorn" (Lyons & Burford, 1992) denouncing certain biotechnology "advances" was received with horror by food technologists. In a panicked response to this release and to the important trend of simplifying agricultural production that will not go away, an article called "Activists Groups Twist Sustainable Agriculture" appeared in Food Technology (April, 1993). Author Ellen Brooks states erroneously that, "Sustainable agriculture is more than a farming philosophy advocating crop rotation and reduced use of pesticides. The movement as Fox describes it seeks to eliminate the contemporary luxuries of meat consumption and modern medicine." She is putting together different, unrelated political movements that frighten food scientists and she is damning them all at once. So I guess we can lump all food scientists into one category without worry...

Food scientists traditionally panic at anything that might change the current way of doing things. I saw this attitude throughout my tenure in a Food Science department. Nobody wants to hear anything which might challenge the teachings they absorbed as children, in college or even in graduate school. Maybe they're afraid? Maybe they think the mind is saturated after "X" amount of learning? I don't know why such resistance exists. Everyone appears to have a maximum tolerance level for new information. It is unfortunate, because if we keep learning, we better ourselves and those around us. Don't be like these intellectually rigid professors. Don't stick your head in the sand; your life might depend on something you hear **after** you think you know everything there is to know.

In 1995, the EPA announced its intention to reduce pesticide use by 66 - 75% by the end of 1996. This suggestion was met with such vigorous opposition that it has not been heard since the first few announcements. I am sure there are those in the EPA that are trying to get this passed through the legislature, but it may be an uphill battle.

A Major Pesticide Tragedy
One of the most unsung, unconsidered tragedies of the overzealous use of pesticides is the loss of beneficial insects. While being threatened by encroachment on their habitat, the destruction of forests, pollution, and even those crummy backyard bug zappers (that never kill mosquitoes, just good insects!), insects are being reduced in greater numbers then imaginable.

"Why should I care?" you ask. "There are millions of them compared to us. And they can live through any disaster..." Well, almost any disaster except human ignorance. Case in point: there were 5 million acres of tallgrass prairie (a major butterfly habitat and feeding ground) in Iowa when the settlers first arrived there. Now there are only 200 acres, and they're all broken into bits and pieces. And it's not the millions of insects of any one species that are decimated; it's the **different species** themselves! Sure there are millions of mosquitoes, roaches, and ants that might be considered undesirable. But when we go to kill them, we are killing other beneficial insects as well as ourselves.

So how does this affect food? I'm glad you asked. Butterflies, bees, beetles, and all the other small animals (Yes, they are biologically classified as members of the Animal Kingdom) are irreplaceable as pollinators of all of our food. Apples, peaches, almonds, blueberries, cranberries, squash, cherries, honey, and dozens of other cash crops are threatened by the loss of beneficial insects through human stupidity with pesticides. It is now so bad that some farmers in Texas, Illinois and Washington have to pay to have thousands of bees trucked into their fields and returned back to their pesticide-free homes after each season in order to have any crop at all.

Crop Fertilization
Why do plants need these insects? Well, it's like this. Plants are fixed in one spot; where we plant them. They're not going anywhere. But they need to produce fruit. Just like we create babies, plants need an egg and a sperm in order to make an embryo (a baby fruit). And just like in human fertilization, it's the sperm that does the traveling and the plant egg that waits. It's kind of hard when you're stuck in one place to go and get a member of the opposite sex to fertilize you. Some plants, like corn, have solved this problem by being monecious, or having both sexes present on each plant. That's what the silk on the corn is for; it provides the sperm, and with the help of the wind, sometimes

fertilizes the female portion of the corn. It's a darn good thing because, as I said before, corn is one of the most heavily pesticided grains and many insects could never survive out in a commercial cornfield.

Other crops are not so fortunate and cannot rely on the wind or rain to supply them with appropriate sperm. These plants have separate female and male individual plants. No matter how close together they are planted, fertilization cannot occur without insects. The male component of fertilization, in order to create most fruits and vegetables, must ride on an insect proboscis or insect legs. It then must be delivered to the appropriate flowering female at the right time.

Another example of how precipitously insect life and fertilization of our crops are linked comes from Time magazine™ reporter Christopher Hallowell in a story about the new book "The Forgotten Pollinators" (Buchmann and Nabhan, 1997). In this article it explains how the "...lowbush blueberry harvest in New Brunswick, Canada, declined by 75% from the previous year after nearby conifer forests were sprayed with pesticides that wiped out the bees that pollinate the blueberries." Further south, Mexico has few environmental controls and allows pesticides to be sprayed willy-nilly. We might be able to ignore it because "it's some other country", but ask anyone on the border of Texas and Mexico about the effects that cross over into the U.S. and you'll get a disturbing story. And you will probably eat some Mexican produce yourself this week; it's in lots of frozen and prepared foods.

Pesticides
To Wage War

1)   Ask at your grocer, "Do you have organic produce?"

2)   Tell your grocer the specific type of produce (apples, bananas, etc.) you want to purchase as organic.

3)   Ask at your favorite restaurant, "Do you cook with organic produce?"

4)   Look for certification on the labels, either COFA (In California), NOFA (In the Northeast) or from the comparable organization in your area.

5)   Find local farmers and show them the potential benefits of going organic (like being able to charge more for a premium quality product).

6)   If you teach, tell all of your pupils about the advantages of organic produce.

7)   Buy products from manufacturers who use only organic produce, like Amy's™ frozen entrees.

Chapter 23
FOOD ADDITIVES

What is a Food Additive?

Anything added to whole food can be considered an additive. Sugar, for example, is an additive in applesauce. When we speak of additives, though, we are more concerned with unusual compounds, especially those that have been synthesized by man. Direct Additives are intentionally added, like sweeteners (sucralose, saccharin, and aspartame). Indirect Additives can be substances that unintentionally get into the food through the processing of the product.

Vitamins are even considered additives in certain foods like flour and rice. Breakfast cereals sell themselves on their additives or vitamin inclusions. "Smarmy Toasties have 100% of 20 Vitamins and Minerals!" Bioavailability notwithstanding, such cereals may hold potential dangers for us with their additive vitamins.

Food additives are used because they impart certain desirable characteristics to a product. Food scientists might determine that a product needs to be a dark cherry red, taste particularly sour, feel like a fat-containing food, or have some other property in order to sell well. They will then find any substance to do the trick. After they determine its success at effecting the changes necessary, they consider its regulatory control. "Can we use it?" is the operative question. Lastly they consider its disease or cancer-causing potential, a major annoyance to food scientists. This is why you, the consumer, as the last bastion of "So what does this do for me?"

need to keep yourself informed. (See the discussion of Red Dye #2 in Chapter 18, Tip #6.)

If a substance is added to a food for a purpose, it is called a Direct Additive. Sweeteners like sucralose and aspartame are considered direct additives. If a substance is not meant to be a part of the formulation of a food, it is an Indirect Additive. Among indirect additives are substances that migrate from the packaging into the food. Cereal manufacturers count on this. BHT was found to cause cancer in certain laboratory studies in the 1970's. The public fear and outcry all but removed it from highly consumed foods. Everything but removed it. When you read "BHT added to packaging", the statement is telling you in a subtle way that it is not in your cereal. The truth is that it migrates into foods from packaging; especially into fatty foods. In fact there are lots of issues with packaging and heavy metals and other toxic or carcinogenic materials. This is one of the reasons, for example, when you get pizza and try to keep your pizza warm or reheat it, you should never do it in the cardboard container.

Additives are used for a variety of reasons. Among the reasons for using additives are product consistency or mouthfeel, for fortification, to maintain taste, to prevent bacterial or fungal growth, to help bread or cakes rise, or to enhance flavor or color. Additives are not new, just more sophisticated than they used to be. Throughout history, additives like salt, sugar, vinegar, and other spices have been used to preserve foods.

Regulation and Approval of Additives

The Food, Drug and Cosmetic (FD&C) Act was designed in 1958 to require FDA approval for any food additive. It hinges mostly upon the way the additive will be used. This is because the government feels, according to the FDA pamphlet "Food

Additives", that "the absolute safety of any substance can never be proven". More important than chemical toxicity and cancer-causing capability, is how much of the substance the average person will consume.

This shift in thinking from "Is it toxic or carcinogenic?" to "But how much of it will the average Joe really get?" compromises our health. I feel that the average consumer should not have to dig desperately for the facts about their food additives, as so many mothers of allergic children have had to do to prevent shock or serious problems in their children. We are all able to decide our own tolerance to risk, if we know what we are consuming.

One of the issues in this FD&C Act of 1958 was that all major additives used up to then were "grandfathered". This meant that all compounds found to be Generally Recognized As Safe (GRAS) were allowable in food forever.

This also meant that compounds like nitrates (potassium and sodium nitrate) were forever allowed to be used in processed meats. These nitrates keep ham pink and sausage reddish. They are implicated as cancer-causing compounds (especially for stomach cancer) in several studies, including the major study of additives performed on an unwitting U.S. public before 1958. Yes, we were guinea pigs then and we're guinea pigs today. By only concerning themselves with the use of products and not whether we should even allow such chemicals in our food, the food scientists are risking more than they have a right to.

The Most Frequently Used Food Additives

Sugar
Salt
Corn Syrup
Dextran Mono- or Di- glycerides
Modified Food Starch

Polysaccharides (Modified Starches)

Polysaccharides have three main functions in foods: to provide structure; to add fiber; and to add calories. Of these, gums and hydrocolloids are most often used in salad dressing and ice cream. CarboxyMethylCellulose (CMC) and Ethyl Cellulose (EC) are the most common.   CMC in ice cream prevents a excessive crystallization during freeze-thaw cycles.   Pectin and starch are also used. Polysaccharides hold water and provide a food with "mouthfeel" and texture similar to that found in more fatty food.

Phenolics

The four major GRAS antioxidants for food are phenolic compounds with great antioxidant capabilities in your food. Several years ago, jokes were made about long lasting, well-preserved corpses unearthed long after burial. It was suggested that all these preservatives in our food made the bodies last longer. If care is taken to insure that antioxidants are not oxidized before we ingest them, it could help preserve us before we go. But if not, we could be killing ourselves with these GRAS antioxidants long before our time.

The four compounds are:

- **BHA** - Butylated hydroxyanisol; used in animal fat. Look for it in your cereals (and cereal packaging) as well.

- **BHT** - Butylated hydroxy toluene; used in animal fat.

- **TBHQ** - Used in vegetable oil

- **Propyl gallate** - Used in vegetable oil

Natural Antioxidants

All are both metal chelators and free radical scavengers. This is part of their antioxidant capabilities. Once again, they will work to destroy you if you get them oxidized or added (as additives) to foods.

- **Alpha-tocopherol**
- **Turmeric**
- **Rosemary**
- **Green tea**
- **EDTA**

Antioxidants in food (Pro-oxidants for you)

Ascorbic Acid-Vitamin C
Alpha Tocopherol-Vitamin E
Beta Carotene-ProVitamin A
Butylated Hydroxyanisole (BHA)
Butylated Hydroxytoluene (BHT)

Synergists

These stop initiation of lipid oxidation, repair phenolic antioxidants by adding oxygen to them, and are used in conjunction with other additives.

- **Phosphoric acid** - Found in cheese, powdered food, cereal, and baked foods, it serves as an emulsifier, chelating agent, and acidulant.

- **Citric acid** - In ice cream, candy, soda, it is used as a chelating agent, acidulant, and an antioxidant in food. Sodium citrate is the most common form.

- **Ascorbic acid** - Helps dry sausage products and ham maintain their pink color. Protects against nitrosamine formation from the nitrate in such products, but in so doing may become a pro-oxidant in your body.

Thickeners

- **Alginate** - Used in canned frosting and dairy products like heavy cream, alginate is derived from seaweed. It stabilizes beer foam and thickens other types of acidic foods.

- **Carrageenan** - Another seaweed derivative, this may be potentially harmful to the colon in large amounts. It is used in ice cream and other foods that need thickening.

- **Corn Syrup** - Corn is the most heavily pesticided grain according to a report out of Cornell University in 1988. It has always concerned me that there might be residue or harmful defects in the chemical composition of the corn syrup. It is used as a cheap filler and thickener in everything! It is in every type of food you can think of. Beware.

- **Gelatin** - Derived from cow bone marrow, it caused a fuss recently, when a vegetarian ate at a Wendy's™ restaurant and discovered gelatin in the dressing on the Veggie Pita. There might be concern over all cow (and eventually other animal) products if analogs or relatives of Mad Cow Disease make it into our herds. Don't think there isn't trouble waiting down the road. There is.

Flavor Enhancers

Flavor enhancers do not have a characteristic taste or aroma of their own, but have the ability to magnify whatever flavor you combine them with. Foods with flavor enhancers include canned vegetables, processed meats, oriental foods and soups, gravies and mixes. Flavor enhancers can be used to modify a flavor as well.

- **Hydrolyzed vegetable protein (HVP)**
- **Monosodium Glutamate (MSG)**
- **Disodium Inosinate**
- **Disodium Guanylate**

Acidity Regulators

- **Lactic acid** - In cheese, frozen desserts, Spanish olives and summer sausage.

- **Phosphoric acid/phosphates** - Found in soda, it is thought to interfere with calcium absorption if ingested in large amounts.

- **Citric acid/Sodium citrate**

Sweetners

Nutritive sweeteners are those which the body can break down and absorb as nutrients. Non-nutritive sweeteners are those which are not broken down in the body, but instead pass through or are absorbed relatively unchanged.

Nutritive Sweeteners

- **Lactose / Milk Sugar** - In breakfast pastry and whipped cream, lactose is also known as common milk sugar and produces gas and discomfort in those who can't tolerate it.

- **Invert sugar / Sucrose / Table Sugar** - In candy, soda, cookies, pastries, cakes and many products, invert sugar is sucrose that has been broken into its two simple sugars, glucose (dextrose) and fructose.

- **Dextrose / Glucose / Confectioners Sugar** - In bread it turns brown when heated. It is also used to dust gum. It readily combines with amino acids like Lysine to complete the Maillard browning (non-enzymatic browning) reaction. This is also called Glycosylation or Carmelization.

- **Fructose / aka Fruit Sugar** - In the Carbohydrates chapter you will find a discussion about fructose and its presence in fruit. It is one of several "Fruit Sugars" including Sucrose, Glucose and others. It is put into foods as a "Natural" sweetener, though any of the sugars could be considered natural. Do not be fooled either by the turbinado sugar in the market. Sugar is sugar.

- **HFCS / High Fructose Corn Syrup** - High Fructose Corn Syrup came into popularity due to a natural disaster in the sugar cane fields about 20 years ago. There was a loss of sugar cane due to pathogen ingression of a fungal disease. This happened with the coffee plants in Sri Lanka years later. In this case, sugar production dropped off and prices soared. Manufacturers ran for the exit as quickly as they could. The result was a big market for HFCS, and nearly all of our processed foods contain some. In Chapter 22 on pesticides, I stated my concerns with pesticided corn and corn products and our inability to avoid them. There's corn product in your cocoa, ice cream, frozen dinners, drink mixes and juices, soups and salad dressings, etc.

- **Sorbitol / Mannitol / Sugar Alcohols** - In gum and candy, these sweeteners have a surprise waiting for those who eat too much of them: diarrhea. These are indigestible carbohydrates like the sugars stachyose and raffinose in beans and bean products. Mannitol is used in limited quantities for specific applications, like the dusting of chewing gum. Sorbitol is used as the main sweetener in some candies and gums.

Non-Nutritive Sweeteners
- **Saccharin**
- **Cyclamate**
- **Aspartame**

Emulsifiers

- Lecithin - Lecithin is also known as a phospholipid and an emulsifier. Its other name is Phosphatidylcholine (see the Lipids discussion in Chapter 6). It is used to thicken and maintain texture in many foods like ice cream.

- **Polysorbate 80**

- **Sorbitan Monostearate**

- **Mono and Diglycerides**

Flavorants

- **Vanilla**

- **Vanillin**

Antimicrobial Agents

Antimicrobial agents are useful for preventing the normal decay of foodstuffs, and prolonging the shelflife of foods. In some cases their antimicrobial tendencies include direct mutation of bacterial, fungal, or viral DNA. There could be a danger to our cells as well if we ingest too much food with these antimicrobial mutagens. We might become victims of unwelcome mutagenic events.

- **Heptyl paraben**
- **Sodium chloride**
- **Sodium nitrite/nitrate**
- **Sodium benzoate**
- **Calcium propionate**
- **Sulfur dioxide/ Sodium bisulfite**
- **Sodium propionate**

Stabilizers / Thickeners

Found in baked goods and frozen desserts, these thickeners and texturizers support the structure of a fatty substance like cream without adding fat. They are very useful in the formulation of smooth, low-fat products. Pectin is used to congeal jams and jellies, except for apple jelly because apples have so much natural pectin they don't need it.

- **Glycerin**
- **Gum**
- **Pectin**
- **Propylene glycol**
- **Hydrogenated vegetable oil**
- **Sodium carboxymethylcellulose**

Food Additives
To Wage War

1) Choose whole foods - these have no additives!

2) Avoid foods containing nitrates, including beef jerky, sausage, and ham.

3) Eat foods that are low in refined sugars.

4) Look at the additives listed on the packages of the foods that you eat. Review this chapter and determine what you will not accept.

5) Avoid foods with sulfites such as dried fruits (e.g., apricots) or red wine.

CAMOUFLAGE

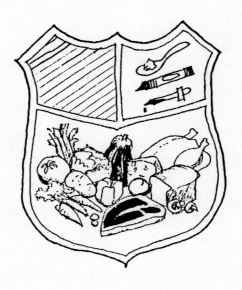

Chapter 24
FLAVORS AND COLORS

Flavors

Flavor is the sensation of a foodstuff that comes to us as a combination of taste and smell. It is a very complex sensation. There are over 4000 chemicals that are components of different flavors. If we were to do a taste test, one of the hundreds of components of coffee flavor might hit you as the true roast flavor of coffee and it might leave me cold.

But the chart of Typical Flavors and Scents on the next page shows that the average person identifies 2-Furylmethanethiol as the essence of coffee. This tells manufacturers of coffee-flavored substances to find and use this volatile chemical, if they cannot use actual coffee in their product. Another component in coffee, trigonelline, decomposes during roasting to give off pyrroles and pyridines (volatile chemical components). These, along with other compounds, are the reason you should "wake up and smell the (antioxidants in your) coffee". These compounds degrade quite quickly, though, and a reheated cup of coffee might do you more harm than good as the good compounds have been volatilized or oxidized.

In Chapter 13, we discussed Mad Cow Disease and recommended you not dust your roses. This is because the rose dust is made of ground up cattle bones, which can be inhaled through your nose and into your brain through a process called reverse axonal transport. What reverse axonal transport might just effect with your coffee is the transport of these coffee volatiles into your brain. Amazing, but potentially true. So mind what you sniff.

Flavors are used to make food desirable and palatable. Food that you'd normally eat would be offensive without any of the flavor components you expect. I'll never forget the time, at the college dining hall, that I tried what I knew was macaroni and cheese. It looked like macaroni and cheese, smelled somewhat like macaroni and cheese, so I ate it. It turned out to be a bizarre type of noodle kugel. I'll never forget my horrified reaction to the sweet, made-with-vanilla-cake-mix entree. It doesn't sound half bad as I describe it here, but my taste buds were horrified. It's all in the expectation. If the flavor isn't right, we don't eat it. (Except for the unfortunate man discussed in the Chapter 13. Whoops. I'll let you read it for yourself.)

The making of black tea, an antioxidant carrying food (see chapter 15), starts with the oxidation of phenolic compounds in the green or original tea leaves. This oxidation creates an orangeish color and the brisk taste of the newly formed theaflavins. This is one of the few cases that flies in the face of my simple antioxidant theory; that once a food is oxidized, it will cause you potential cancerous harm. Antioxidant compounds in tea, known as catechins, are oxidized to form other antioxidant compounds known as theaflavins and thearubigens.

Flavors are largely determined by three parameters:

5%   Basic taste sensation
90% Olfactory (Smell)
5%   Mouthfeel sensation

Odor accounts for 90% of all tastes. The ability to smell is essential to any exercise involving food. There are seven primary odors according to the site-fitting theory listed below. The sensation of these separate odor components depends upon a combination of their shape, size and electrical charge.

The Seven Primary Odors

Camphor   Ethereal
Musk   Floral
Mint   Pungent
Putrid

We have specific areas of the tongue and specific taste buds that respond to the five basic tastes. The diagram of the tongue shows a chevron of Bitter sensation in the back of the tongue as well as a Sweet section in the front, and Sour and Salty on the sides.

The Five Basic Tastes

Salt   Sweet
Sour   Bitter
Umami

Three examples of taste buds that can be specific to taste sensations are fungiform (which look like mushrooms), foliate (which look like tree trunks), and circumvallate (which have an indentation around the outside). The circumvallate are largely for bitter sensations, while the foliate serve as sour detectors.

The Tongue

The tongue is the organ of taste. It has small bumps all over the surface called taste buds. There are four basic kinds of taste buds:

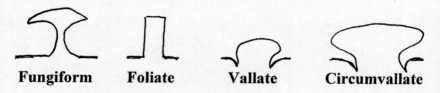

Fungiform   **Foliate**   **Vallate**   **Circumvallate**

The Tongue

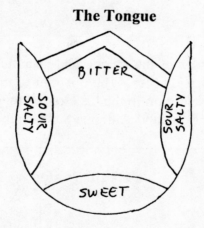

Taste is sensed through 4 of the **12 Cranial Nerves** that connect your sensations to your brain. **The Trigeminal (the 5th)** is largely responsible for the response to texture and mouthfeel in foods. **The Vagus (the 10th)** enervates the palate (the roof of your mouth) and your esophagus. This allows the Vagus to participate in texture assessment as well. The **Chordatympani (the 7th)** enervates the front of the tongue and assesses sweet, sour, and salty. The **Glossopharyngeal (the 9th)** responds to or enervates the circumvallate and foliar papillae (taste buds). The Glossopharyngeal nerve is therefore responsible for a response to bitter tastes at the chevron of taste buds at the back of the tongue. The gag reflex, in response to poisonous or bitter substances, is initiated at this site.

The Umami taste sensation is a fairly recent inclusion because it has been determined by Japanese and U.S. scientists to be responded to by a separate function that is stimulated by Far Eastern foods.

Bitter taste buds on the back of the tongue serve a necessary function. It is thought that they are responsible for the "gag" reflex whenever we encounter anything poisonous. The necessity of this function is obvious because most medicines are bitter, as are poisonous plant alkaloids we might have, at one time in human history, encountered in the wild. I'm sure this contributes to our inability to ingest pills without thinking hard about it or floating them in drinks of water.

How Companies Know Your Tastes

Sensory Analysis is the study of likes and dislikes of product consumers. All companies do some form of analysis of the appreciation of their product. They may call it a focus group study, a home use test (HUT), or an analysis of consumer satisfaction. Anyway you look at it, sensory analysis plays a large part in corporate America.

Some sensory analysis, like that which I personally performed at a large corporation, is designed to see just how cheaply a company can skimp on ingredients and whether the average consumer can tell the difference. This is the unfortunate use of sensory analysis; there are better uses, such as in product development. When products are first being developed, the prototype must be tested by scientists in-house and eventually consumer tested.

Take this test. Go and get a favorite cracker and try these tests. Take a bite of the cracker and evaluate it. If one bite isn't enough, rinse your mouth with water and take another bite. Place a slash across the lines below, in the appropriate place, to indicate where you feel the characteristics of the sample lie.

The characteristics here may not be representative of the food you chose, but we'll address that later. Just try and evaluate.

Sweet--Not Sweet

Soft---Crunchy

Aromatic--Bland

How did your cracker do? Was it more Aromatic or Bland? Did you have someone else give their opinion too? Was it the same as yours? Not enough descriptive words? Hard to find the taste or smell that is requested? You'll find sensory departments in all food companies working long hours to refine tests to ask what is needed and to be understandable to you - the consumer.

At the end of this chapter you will find more sophisticated sensory tests for your own experimentation. Use them with friends, classes, kids, or just for fun for yourself.

Typical Flavors and Scents / Underlying Chemical Compounds	
Mint	Menthol / Menthone
Licorice	Anisaldehyde / Anethole
Pineapple	Ethyl Valerate / Ethyl Pelargonate
Banana	Isoamyl Acetate
Pine	Pinene / Terpene
Almond	Benzaldehyde
Orange	Limonene
Vanilla	Vanillin
Cinnamon	Cinnamic Aldehyde
Nutmeg	Eugenol / Terpenes
Cloves	Eugenol
Coffee	2-Furylmethanethiol
Tomato	cis-2-hexenal
Cucumber	2-nonenal / 2,6-nonadienal
Grapefruit	Nootkatone / 1-p-menthene-8-thiol
Lemon	Citral

Colors

Why do we see color in pigments? It turns out that it is a function of the internal bonding (conjugated bonds absorb and show color more) and the capturing and bending of light of a given pigment. This light is bent in such a way that the rods and cones in our eyes can discern one color from another and black from white. We use color to make decisions in very subtle ways that we may not even be aware of.

A now famous sensory experiment was performed in which several consumer volunteers were asked to assess the sweetness of an ice cream sherbet. They were given identical portions of the same lime sherbet on two separate occasions and asked their opinion. The only difference was that one was colored purplish and one colored light green. The participants could identify the lime flavor

75% of the time in the green colored one, but only 47% of the time in the purple sherbet! The color influenced the flavor. Or more precisely, our perception of the flavor.

The red color of a cooked lobster is due to its normal green/blue color turning into astaxanthin, a red pigment related to beta-carotene. The red of red bell pepper is from a different red compound, capxanthin. The orange-brown color used in self-tanning formulas is called canthaxanthin, another beta-carotene related pigment.

Strawberry red color is from pelargonoidin-3-glucoside, a flavonoid derivative. Once again, the flavonoids are both anti- and pro-oxidants in different situations. Another flavonoid that has great antioxidant potential is Quercetin. It provides the yellowish to muddy gray colors of canned asparagus, onions, the bark of douglas fir, and mushrooms. A very powerful antioxidant, we have to assume that the opposite is also true if you eat old, or temperature abused samples of those foods.

The HEME Groups

One of my pigment theories is that the structures called "hemes", "porphyrin rings" or "tetrapyrroles" that hold other small molecules onto themselves to create color are all interrelated and possibly exchangeable. This tetrapyrrole molecule is so large and elaborate that there are really just four major types that we ingest: hemoglobin (in the blood of other animals, or what we call gravy); myoglobin (in the muscle meat of other animals); Vitamin B-12 (from our intestinal microbes); and chlorophyll (in all green plants). Hemoglobin has an iron molecule at its center, and it provides the color of oxygenated and deoxygenated blood, red and blue respectively.

Myoglobin also has an iron center and it changes the color of the meat after slaughter. In the supermarket packages you can see red, purplish, and brown meat. These are the results of three states of myoglobin; oxymyoglobin, myoglobin, and metmyoglobin, respectively. The addition of Nitric Oxide to pork/ham upon heating forms another version of myoglobin that is pink, nitrosohemochrome. This is the typical cured meat color.

Chlorophyll is nearly identical to both myoglobin and hemoglobin, but has a phytol tail. I think this lends credence to vegetarianism as evolutionarily designed. We don't need hemoglobin or myoglobin from other animals if we have chlorophyll. Chlorophyll supplies plants with their green color due to a magnesium (instead of iron) molecule in its center. There is some sort of grand design in having the identical complex molecule found in both plants and animals. It lends even more credence to the fact that vegetarians are not missing out on anything nutritional by not eating meat.

The Major Pigment Groupings In Plants

Flavonoids-Benzopyran Derivatives
Anthocyanins-Benzopyran Derivatives
Carotenoids-Isoprenoid Units
Chlorophyll-Tetrapyrrole
Polyphenols-Melanoidins

Corporate Sensory Tests

Appearance Test

This test can be used for any type of product. Copy this form several times or design your own for fun. This is a good tool to train adults and children in evaluation skills.

Use the test below to determine your evaluation of the appearance of a product. Put a slash through the line between the attributes exactly where you feel a description of that attribute falls.

Example:

Light Blue---/-----Dark Blue

[This person feels that the sample they were given is very dark blue.]

SIZE

Small---Large

Thin--Thick

SHAPE

Flat--Not Flat

Round--Not Round

Square---Not Square

Uniform--Not uniform

Appearance Test

COLOR

Light--Dark

Dull--Bright

Even--Blotchy

SHADES

White--Yellow

Yellow--Green

Pink--Red

Orange--Red

Blue--Green

Purple--Blue

Purple--Pink

TEXTURE

Smooth--Rough

Thin--Thick

Even--Gritty

Gritty--Lumpy

Basic Tastes

The five basic tastes are sweet, salty, sour, bitter and umami. Because Umami is difficult to explain to Western cultures (it is best understood in the Orient) it has been eliminated from this test.

Sweet--Not Sweet

Salty---Not Salty

Sour--Not Sour

Bitter--Not Bitter

Saliva: The Adapting Solution

Saliva contains many compounds including water, amino acids, sugars and salts. Different concentrations of each are present in different people at different times. Typical concentrations in saliva of each of the 4 Basic Tastes are found below.

Typical Salivary Concentrations Of Taste Components	
Sucrose = 0.01 Molar	Acid = 0.001 Molar
Salt = 0.03 Molar	Bitter = 0.0007 Molar

Think of a time when you ate something very sweet, like pancakes and syrup (or even brushed your teeth), and then drank orange juice. The sourness of the juice was readily apparent due to the high sugar content of the saliva. Just as people with a love for salty foods probably have a higher salt concentration in their saliva than others, so do diabetics have a higher concentration of sweetness which prevents their ability to know a sweet food as sweet.

The concentration of bitter is evolutionarily purposeful. Most poisons are bitter. The concentration of bitter is therefore low enough that we might be able to perceive the major plant alkaloids which are poisonous, thus saving our lives.

Basic Chemical Feel

Chemical feel of a substance often comes from the enervation of the trigeminal nerve (one of the twelve cranial, or head nerves) in your mouth. This is not the same as taste because you can have this sensation without tasting anything. It is the cool feel of mint and menthol, the hot of chili peppers, the carbonation of champagne or soda, and the astringency or acidy feel of the tannins in tea, coffee or wine which produce this nerve excitation.

```
Cool----------------------------------------------------------------Not Cool

Hot------------------------------------------------------------------Not Hot

Acidy--------------------------------------------------------------Not Acidy

Flat----------------------------------------------------------------Bubbly
```

Texture Studies

Have you ever eaten a soggy cookie, had milk with lumps in it, or felt unusual sliminess on a product? Your ability to determine texture could save your life! If you've ever had a foreign substance in your food and found it with your tongue or not eaten something that had an unusual texture for that type of food, you have known the power of texture evaluation. While we can't give every possible texture parameter here, you can use this as a general list and design your own tests.

Compression in Mouth

Springy---Not Springy

Slippery---Sticky

Soft---Firm

Cuts easily---Cannot cut

Airy---Compact

Manipulation in Mouth

Small particles---Large

Small # Particles---Many Particles

Clean feel---Mouth coated

Oily---Dry

Adhesive---Easily removed

Crumbles---Breaks large

GUERRILLA TACTICS

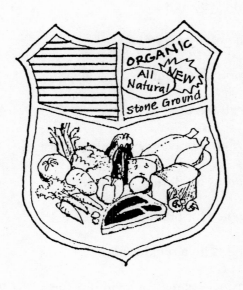

HOW FIT ARE YOU?

Answer "True" or "False" to the following statements. Then rate
yourself using the chart below. *"Aerobics"* means any form of
exercise that really gets your heart going, not just formal classes.

1)	I truly enjoy exercise.	True	False
2)	I walk to get my energy up.	True	False
3)	I do *aerobics* for 20min / 2X a week	True	False
4)	I stretch all the time.	True	False
5)	My life / job involves physical exercise	True	False
6)	I do *aerobics* for 30min / 3X a week	True	False
7)	I do *aerobics* for 60min / 3 +X a week	True	False
8)	I lift weights on a regular basis	True	False
9)	I play physical games or swim for fun	True	False
10)	I tell others of the benefits of exercise.	True	False

To determine your fitness category, add up your score and check the fitness chart below. While this test oversimplifies fitness levels, it reminds us that if we are to wage war against poor health, we must be physically fit. As my favorite television exercise personality, Gilad Janklowitz, says, "If you rest, you rust!"

Question	True	False
1	5 pts	2 pts
2	5 pts	2 pts
3	7 pts	2 pts
4	5 pts	2 pts
5	8 pts	2 pts
6	8 pts	2 pts
7	10 pts	2 pts
8	8 pts	2 pts
9	5 pts	2 pts
10	4 pts	2 pts

[The reason I give 2 points for "False" is that you deserve points for trying this quiz - and not every "False" is detrimental to your fitness level. More important are the "True" answers.]

Scoring	
20-25 points:	You need to get up right now and start exercising, lightly. Consult your physician before starting any exercise program.
26-38 points	This is a good start toward physical health and vigor. Try to keep this level and increase your activity a little all the time.
39-47 points	Excellent effort! Your future health will benefit from your level of exercise.
48-65 points	You're cooking with gas! Keep up the good work!

and I have switched to another cereal. The hard candies that used to be filled with real juice from a major manufacturer now include mostly corn syrup and coloring. They taste like it too. Apple juice is almost always sugar water and a little apple for good luck. Even my dog's biscuits are shrinking! To get around having to give the consumer real good food product, these companies set forth legislation about the Standard of Identity, a way of regulating what can legally be called what.

Abusing the Standard Of Identity - Fat Free Food

"Fat Free" food is technically considered food that has less than approximately 0.8 grams of triglyceride per serving. Does this surprise you? It should. In other words, if you eat 10 small "fat free" cookies you could be eating up to **8 grams of fat!**

How can food manufacturers do this? Well, they have helped define this standard to allow the industry some leeway in creation and production of products. They can legally list the fat per serving as "0 grams" when it is really almost 1 gram. One major manufacturer went so far as to push the limit and make it 1 gram per serving while calling it 0 grams per serving, but they were chastised by the industry and forced to lower the fat to 0.8 grams or remove their "Fat-Free" label.

There is another, more elaborate trick. The definition of "fat" to food manufacturers is "triglyceride". Now, fat is very important in delivering flavor components to your palate, and the food producers all know this. Manufacturers need to use fat in some products to make them taste good. They came up with a clever way around the standard. Since "triglycerides" were not allowed, they use mono- and di-glycerides. Look closely at your labels of, for example, fat-free cakes and cookies. If you look back in the Chapter 6 on fats, you will see that the only difference between a diglyceride and a triglyceride is the removal of one of the fatty acid chains in the triglyceride. The triglyceride could be formed again any number of ways, including sometime after you ingest it. In other words, you are getting fat in your food; it's just a slightly different kind. And this fat can make you fat just like triglycerides can.

To be fair, some makers of fat-free food do not use this rule to their advantage and they try to use other ways to make the flavors come out. But, you need to read the ingredient list on every food to know. Don't forget that raisins and yogurt have fat too! A number of manufacturers of fat-free food use those ingredients as whole foods and it makes the label read better, but there's still fat present.

Buzz Words and Phrases Designed To Fool The Public

100% Pure--Not From Concentrate
A number of fruit juice manufacturers use this phrase. What do you think you'd get if you bought the product labelled with the phrase above? Fresh squeezed juice? Well, O.K., it's not from concentrate...What is "Concentrate"?

"Concentrate" is used to refer to frozen juice that has been concentrated and rehydrated to put in a juice carton. It also refers to the juices you buy and rehydrate. The juice above was not frozen and reconstituted for shipment to your grocer's shelves. No. It was dried into **volatile chemical components,** had other **synthetic chemicals** (like the carcinogenic Limonene) added to it and shipped!

The story behind the juice above is one that has stuck in my craw since I found out about it. I have paid many extra dollars over the years thinking I was getting the best, freshest juice on the market, only to find out that I was drinking dried mixed chemicals with foreign flavor chemicals added to local water! That's right!! As they ship this dried, remixed, and augmented-with-chemical-flavorant powder around the country, it gets rehydrated with whatever water is locally available. There may be nothing wrong with your local water, but nonetheless, I want my water directly from the inside of the orange.

All Natural

We see this designation on at least one package of just about every edible product you can name today. There will always be some version of these products that is *"All Natural"* or *"Natural"* or *"Nature-Made"*. You get the idea. The problem with this designation is that **it means absolutely nothing** !!! How many of us have opted for the "Natural" ice cream instead of the ice cream that doesn't say it's "Natural"? I used to tell my students that all it means is that, well, because it's cold and made with milk and sugar, *"Naturally*, it's ice cream!" There are no federal guidelines regarding *"Natural"* as a designation. The only true information you are legally entitled to is the list of ingredients, and I suggest you look at them carefully.

Stone Ground

Stone Ground, Whole Grain, Wheat Flour... All of these designations are not telling you exactly what you need to hear, which is "Whole Wheat" or "Whole Rice", etc. *Stone Ground* is really meaningless when it comes to the healthiness and fiber content of your bread. You need to know if your bread includes the whole grain and only the word, "Whole", in the ingredient listing will give you this information.

Chemical Free

Ah, my favorite. This designation acknowledges the phobia that underlines so much of what we search for in terms of product safety. *Chemical Free.* Just the placement of that evil word next to the ultimate good word gives us a warm feeling. Well I have some bad news for those of you who look for these products.

There is no such thing! The entire earth, the atmosphere, your clothes, your dog, your trees and you, are just creative blobs of chemicals! That's right. Your *Chemical Free* moisturizer is just another blob of chemicals in a jar. All we see and are and hope to have is made of chemicals.

Granted, some chemicals are worse than others, but you won't find the safer things necessarily in the health food store. In fact, it is a creative minefield. Pick the wrong thing and your health can blow up in your face! How about some Ma Huang or Ephedra tea? It causes your heartbeat to accelerate. One small, weak cup won't hurt you unless you're sensitive, so how about a little more for "herbal ecstasy"? One confirmed teenage death from too much should have been enough of a warning, but it wasn't. Be careful with herbal preparations.

There are unusual, untested, and potentially dangerous supplements in the health food stores. There is, for example, an *all natural, chemical free, organic* hair dye that contains a chemical that is so toxic it is a guaranteed spermicide. I am continually amazed at the food and supplements that are available. Nearly all of the supplements in my local health food store have <u>no expiration date</u> on them! This means that they could have expired in 1979! Who knows? In the Antioxidants and Vitamins section I've explained that old vitamins can give you cancer! Be sure that you only buy <u>dated</u> food and vitamins!

Tricks of the Trade
To Wage War

1) Look at all packages - read everything.

2) Contact manufacturers of shrinking products, substituted ingredients, and changing tastes. Ask them why!

3) Talk to your local congressperson if you feel you're being cheated. A lot can be accomplished at the grass-roots level (look at the cereal industry fiasco in 1997).

4) Buy alternative products from caring manufacturers to show your displeasure with companies that act underhandedly.

<u>APPENDIX I</u>

<u>How Fit Are You?</u>

HOW FIT ARE YOU?

Answer "True" or "False" to the following statements. Then rate yourself using the chart below.

1) Exercise relaxes me.   True   False

2) I often walk or hike for recreation.   True   False

3) At least twice a week, I exercise   True   False
    vigorously for 20 minutes.

4) I regularly do yoga or stretching   True   False
    exercises.

5) My work includes heavy lifting   True   False
    and vigorous physical exercise.

6) I participate in vigorous recreational   True   False
    sports about three times a week.

7) I participate in vigorous recreational   True   False
    sports about once a week.

8) Given a choice, I will always take   True   False
    the stairs over the elevator.

9) Most of my exercise is gardening   True   False
    or light household chores.

10) I usually walk to work or to shop.   True   False

To determine your fitness category, add up your score and check the fitness chart below. While this test oversimplifies fitness levels, it reminds us that if we are to wage war against poor health, we must be physically fit. As my favorite television exercise personality, Gilad Janklowitz, says, "If you rest, you rust!"

Question	True	False
1	5 pts	2 pts
2	5 pts	2 pts
3	7 pts	2 pts
4	4 pts	2 pts
5	8 pts	2 pts
6	10 pts	2 pts
7	4 pts	2 pts
8	4 pts	2 pts
9	3 pts	2 pts
10	4 pts	2 pts

[The reason I give 2 points for "False" is that you deserve points for trying this quiz - and not every "False" is detrimental to your fitness level. More important are the "True" answers.]

Scoring	
20-25 points:	You need to get up right now and start exercising, lightly. Consult your physician before starting any exercise program.
26-38 points	This is a good start toward physical health and vigor. Try to keep this level and increase your activity a little all the time.
39-47 points	Excellent effort! Your future health will benefit from your level of exercise.
48-54 points	You're cooking with gas! Keep up the good work!

APPENDIX II

Rating TV Fitness Programs

RATING TV FITNESS PROGRAMS

If you are considering starting an exercise program, you may want to start at home. Gyms can be intimidating places where really buffed, fit individuals go to display their physiques as they get even better. Couch potatoes can feel discouraged at first. The next best thing is to get videos or watch any of the various exercise programs at home. Once you reach your desired level of fitness, you can go strut your stuff at the gym and work out with the best.

You may also find that gym workouts are very much more intense than you are used to. There are beginning classes for new exercisers, but they are taught by very fit and intensely exercising instructors. They can shame you into doing more reps than you should, bending farther than you should, and even doing exercises that will hurt you. You need to start slowly and build. Do not join a gym after years of inactivity and just jump right in. You will get hurt. If you don't hurt lower back muscles (a common problem), then your heart will be straining from the new, active you.

Get up right now and find some exercise or recreational activity that you enjoy. Just go slowly until you are really fit for intensity. Television exercise shows are usually only a half an hour and most offer a good mixed workout. If you're not home for them, get their videos or tape them for later use.

Quality Ratings
A = Excellent; B = Good; C = Fair; D = Poor; F = Really Poor

Intensity Ratings
1 = Very Low; for beginners ------- 10 = High Impact; very intense

Basic Training with Ada Janklowitz

Music appropriate	B
Easy to follow	A
Gradual changes	A
Instructor has rhythm	B
Uses entire body	A
Considers older or handicapped	B
Kid-friendly	A

Ada has basic moves, some yoga, and good but easy stretching. Very good for beginners or those returning to exercise. The exercises are easy to follow.
Intensity = 4

Victoria's Body Shop

Music appropriate	A
Easy to follow	B
Gradual changes	B
Instructor has rhythm	A
Uses entire body	B
Considers older or handicapped	C
Kid-friendly	B

Victoria has great presence, enthusiasm, and a good sense of dance and rhythm. It is fun to try, if difficult to follow sometimes.
Intensity = 6

Perfect Parts

Music appropriate	C
Easy to follow	B
Gradual changes	B
Instructor has rhythm	D
Uses entire body	C
Considers older or handicapped	D
Kid-friendly	C

Perfect Parts has three exercisers who work at various ability levels. None of the participants has a lot of rhythm sense or understanding of their audience's abilities. It is easy to follow. Intensity = 3 - 4

Get Fit with Denise Austin

Music appropriate	B
Easy to follow	C
Gradual changes	B
Instructor has rhythm	C
Uses entire body	B
Considers older or handicapped	B
Kid-friendly	B

Denise has a wonderful attitude and many people I've talked to, love her. But sometimes her motions are too large and you might get hurt if you don't understand how much more fit she is than you. She is in amazing shape for a mother of two and is very credible. Intensity = 5 - 7

Bodies In Motion with Gilad Janklowitz

Music appropriate	B
Easy to follow	A
Gradual changes	A
Instructor has rhythm	A
Uses entire body	A
Considers older or handicapped	A
Kid-friendly	A

The absolute best fitness show on television. Gil combines his muscle knowledge as an Olympic athlete with an understanding of his varied audience. Exercises are designed for low, high, or middle impact. Moves are carefully controlled as not to hurt you and his changes are easy and understandable. Gil considers exercises for the elderly, handicapped, and the very young, all of whom he has on his show. A great motivator, he hooked me years ago as I turned on the television, went to the fridge with my cup of coffee, and he said, "Get over here! Put that coffee down, get out of the refrigerator and come exercise with me!" How did he know?
Intensity = 3 - 8 (You can choose your own!)

The Body Shop(Crunch) with Kelsie Daniels

Music appropriate	A
Easy to follow	A
Gradual changes	A
Instructor has rhythm	A
Uses entire body	B
Considers older or handicapped	C
Kid-friendly	B

Kelsie has got the most exciting music and dance exercise show on today. She is easy to follow and enthusiastic enough to make you want to get up and join her, even though the moves may be tricky for non-hiphoppers. She carefully tells you when she's about to change her motions and has a whole posse behind her.
Intensity = 6-7

Gotta Sweat with Cory Everson

Music appropriate	C
Easy to follow	B
Gradual changes	B
Instructor has rhythm	D
Uses entire body	C
Considers older or handicapped	C
Kid-friendly	C

Easy winner of the most perfect body on television, Cory is amazing. She understands and knows all of her muscle groups and can tell you the perfect exercise with weights for just about any purpose. Very pleasant, but not really motivating, her rhythm is lacking and many of the lifting exercises are not appropriate for couch potatoes, kids or the handicapped. And who has all those weight machines in their house? I think most people probably watch with free weights and approximate the exercises; a potentially dangerous prospect if you don't know what you're doing.
Intensity = 3-5

APPENDIX III

3- or 6-Day Diet Analysis

USDA FOOD GUIDE PYRAMID

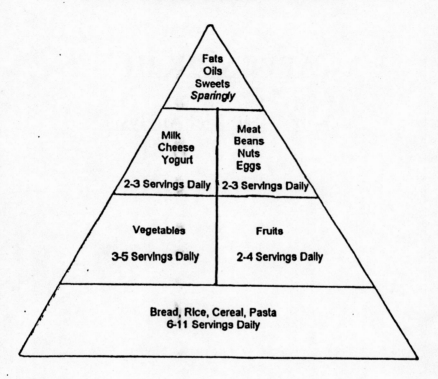

Fats
Oils
Sweets
Sparingly

Milk
Cheese
Yogurt

2-3 Servings Daily

Meat
Beans
Nuts
Eggs

2-3 Servings Daily

Vegetables

3-5 Servings Daily

Fruits

2-4 Servings Daily

Bread, Rice, Cereal, Pasta
6-11 Servings Daily

The USDA Food Guide Pyramid was designed by nutritionists and the United States Department of Agriculture for use in diet evaluation and adjustment. It gives general guidelines as to what are the correct amounts of basic nutrients in a healthy diet. If constructing specific diets is too much for you, just use the pyramid as a guide. If you are eating (approximately) the amounts of each nutrient listed, your diet should be O.K.

3- or 6-Day Diet Record
Step 1 - Setting Up Your Record

How To Create A 3- Or 6-Day Diet Record

1)   Pick any three or six <u>consecutive</u> days, in advance.
2)   Try to use a weekend day attached to two weekdays.
3)   Specifically describe the food you eat.
4)   Don't purposefully eat differently at any time during the recording period.
5)   Be accurate about amounts eaten:
   Use a measuring cup; fill with water then pour in a glass
   Use a measuring cup for dry food; look at on plate
   Use a measuring spoon to test both dry and wet substances
6)   Practice several times with measuring devices for accuracy.
7)   Ask about portion sizes in restaurants.
8)   Write down ABSOLUTELY EVERYTHING - Drinks too!
9)   Don't overestimate or underestimate the food you've eaten.
10)   Keep a pad and pen with you so you get everything eaten.
11)   Butter, mayonnaise, jam, gravy, water, etc. all count!

SAMPLE RECORD

Food Description	Amount	Group	#Servings
Glass of milk	8 oz.	Milk	1
Toast	4oz. slice	Grain	1
(with butter)	1tsp.	Milk	1
Ham slice	8 oz.	Meat	2

Use this as a guide to help you lay out your 3 (or 6) days. Your foods will be different, but you can estimate. *Use this format to do the more accurate 6 Day Diet Analysis as well.*

Step 1 (continued)

YOUR FOOD RECORD----Copy This Form Several Times!

Breakfast and AM snacks

Food Description	Amount	Group	#Servings

Lunch and snacks

Food Description	Amount	Group	#Servings

Dinner and PM snacks

Food Description	Amount	Group	#Servings

Step 2 - Food Groups

There are three tasks you need to complete for Step 2.

Classify food into groups
This can be the most difficult part if you've never done it before, so we'll give you a few examples and tell you the correct food group.

> *An 8 oz. cup of juice = 2 fruit/vegetable servings*
> *Four tablespoons of nut butter = 1 meat group serving*
> *1 tablespoon of butter = Put in "Other" group*
> *1 english muffin (or hamburger bun) = 2 grain servings*
> *1 large bagel = 3 grain servings*
> *Cookies, pie, candy, bacon or chips = "Other" category*
> *2 cups popcorn = 1 Grain serving*
> *1/2 cup pasta or rice = 1 Grain serving*

Count the number of servings from each group
Serving sizes are specific, they are NOT the amount you sat down and ate at a meal! Rather, they are the amounts listed in the Serving Sizes chart on the next page. You must estimate from this chart (or better yet, buy one of those little, inexpensive food guides you see on the check-out line at the supermarket. They are very helpful if you cannot estimate easily). <u>Do not forget to break down combination dishes like pot pie, casseroles, or even hamburgers into their component parts and food groups.</u>

Total up all your food groups. Be careful with your calculations.

Compare number of servings with recommended amounts
Make a note of where you miss the mark. Keep this record handy while you complete the rest of the survey.

The Four Food Group Serving Sizes

MEAT, EGGS, NUTS, SEEDS (3 servings/day)

1.5 cups dry beans   3 oz. meat
0.75 cups of nuts   2 eggs
0.75 cups of seeds (sunflower or sesame)

DAIRY (3 servings/day)

1 cup milk (8oz.)   1 cup yogurt
1.25 oz. cheese   2 cups cottage cheese
2 cups ice cream

FRUIT/VEGETABLE (5 servings/day)

1/2 grapefruit   1/2 cantelope
medium potato   0.5 cup vegetables

GRAIN (6 - 10 servings/day)

1 slice of bread   1/2 bagel
0.5 cup cooked cereal   1 oz. cold cereal

FATS/OILS/SUGAR
(As few as possible; minimum 10 grams/day)

Butter   Olive oil
Canola oil   Mayonnaise
Refined sugar

Step 2

Food Group Servings

Determine the food group, write down the amount you ate, and
then note that amount <u>in serving sizes</u> (use one form per day).

Type of Food	Amount You Ate	Meat	Dairy	Fruit/Veg	Grain	Other
		---------- Number of Serving Sizes ----------				

Totals From Food Groups For 3 or 6 Day Analysis

Enter your daily food group totals on the following table.

Food group:	Meat	Dairy	Fruit/Vegetable	Grain
DAY 1				
DAY 2				
DAY 3				
DAY 4				
DAY 5				
DAY 6				
TOTALS				

Take your Total for each Group and divide by number of days.

EXAMPLE

Grain Group Total = $\dfrac{21.5 \ servings}{6 \ day \ diet}$ = 3.6 servings/Day

So your servings per day were 3.6. The recommended number of servings for the Grain Group is 6 per day. You're close to the recommended minimum amount, so keep it up and increase your intake from this group a little bit.

Servings/Day	MEAT	DAIRY	FRUIT/VEG	GRAIN
Your #				
Recommended #	3	3	5 each	6-10

Step 3 - Nutrient Analysis

Get A Vitamin/Mineral Guide For Whole Foods
In the analysis of vitamins and minerals, it is necessary to obtain a guide that lists the vitamin and mineral content of whole and unprocessed foods. Such a guide need only be one of those small, inexpensive paperbacks you can find on the supermarket checkout line. It is important to get a new guide even if you have an old one lying around, because measurements change over time as do daily requirements. This will allow you to measure the approximate mineral content of all of your unprocessed foods.

Use Package Nutrition Labels For Processed Foods
In obtaining the vitamin/mineral content of your food from the package label, do not forget to multiply or divide by the number of servings that you ate. It may be necessary to estimate the division of the package contents in order to assess your portion.

Add Both Estimates Together For Your Total Intake
Add the vitamin/mineral estimate of the packaged foods together with the whole food estimate of vitamins and minerals to obtain your total intake. Divide the totals by 3 or 6 (depending upon the number of days you ran the diet analysis) for each vitamin or mineral. This will give you an average of your daily intake of these nutrients. Then proceed to the last section to see what action you should take, if any.

Vitamins / Minerals

Vitamins

	A	B-1	B-2	B-6	B-12	Folate	C	D	E	K
Food										
Totals										

Divide these totals by the number of days that you ran your diet
analysis (e.g. 3 or 6) and that will give you correct numbers to
compare to the chart in Section 4.

Minerals

	Ca	Fe	Mg	K	P	Cl	Mn	Se	Zn	Na
Food										
Totals										

Divide these totals by the number of days that you ran your diet analysis (e.g. 3 or 6) and that will give you correct numbers to compare to the chart in Section 4.

Calories/Protein/Carbohydrate/Fat

Calories   Protein (gm)   Carbohydrate (gm)   Fat (gm)

Food

_____

_____

_____

_____

_____

_____

_____

_____

_____

_____

_____

_____

_____

Totals_____

Divide these totals by the number of days that you ran your diet analysis (e.g. 3 or 6) and that will give you correct numbers to compare to the chart in Section 4.

Step 4 - Action For Health

Evaluate the information you have gathered and plan to modify your intake accordingly. You may want to re-evaluate your diet by repeating this diet analysis every 6 months or so to track your nutritional progress.

Food Group Servings

I Consume
Too Much   Too Little   Correct Amount

Fats / Oils / Sweets _____
Meats / Dairy _____
Fruits / Vegetables _____
Grain _____

My Food Group plan of action includes:
Increasing my intake of_____
by_____
Increasing my intake of_____
by_____
Increasing my intake of_____
by_____

Decreasing my intake of_____
by_____
Decreasing my intake of_____
by_____
Decreasing my intake of_____
by_____

<u>Vitamins</u>

I Consume
<u>Too Much   Too Little   Correct Amount</u>

Vitamin A   _____
Vitamin B-1   _____
Vitamin B-2   _____
Vitamin B-3   _____
Vitamin B-6   _____
Vitamin B-12   _____
Folic Acid   _____
Biotin   _____
Vitamin C   _____
Vitamin D   _____
Vitamin E   _____
Vitamin K   _____

My Vitamin plan of action includes:
Increasing my intake of_____
by_____
Increasing my intake of_____
by_____
Increasing my intake of_____
by_____

Decreasing my intake of_____
by_____
Decreasing my intake of_____
by_____
Decreasing my intake of_____
by_____

Minerals
I Consume

	Too Much	Too Little	Correct Amount
Calcium (Ca)			
Iron (Fe)			
Potassium (K)			
Sodium (Na)			
Phosphorus (P)			
Manganese (Mn)			
Magnesium (Mg)			
Selenium (Se)			
Silicon (Si)			
Zinc (Zn)			
Iodine (I)			
Chromium (Cr)			
Chloride (Cl-)			
Copper (Cu)			
Fluoride (F)			
Molybdenum (Mo)			

My Mineral plan of action includes:

Increasing my intake of_____

by_____

Increasing my intake of_____

by_____

Increasing my intake of_____

by_____

Decreasing my intake of_____

by_____

Decreasing my intake of_____

by_____

Decreasing my intake of_____

by_____

Calories/Protein/Carbohydrate/Fat
I Consume

	Too Much	Too Little	Correct Amount
Total Calories			
Protein			
Carbohydrate			
Fat			

My Nutrient plan of action includes:

Increasing my intake of_____

by_____

Increasing my intake of_____

by_____

Increasing my intake of_____

by_____

Decreasing my intake of_____

by_____

Decreasing my intake of_____

by_____

Decreasing my intake of_____

by_____

APPENDIX IV

The Fatty Acids

The Fatty Acids

Name   # Carbons   #C : # Dbl. Bonds   System Name

Saturated Fatty Acids			
Butyric	4	4:0	n-Butanoic
Caproic	6	6:0	n-Hexanoic
Caprylic	8	8:0	n-Octanoic
Capric	10	10:0	n-Decanoic
Lauric	12	12:0	n-Dodecanoic
Myristic	14	14:0	n-Tetradecanoic
Palmitic	16	16:0	n-Hexadecanoic
Stearic	18	18:0	n-Octadecanoic
Arachidic	20	20:0	n-Eicosanoic
Behenic	22	22:0	n-Docosanoic
Lignoceric	24	24:0	n-Tetracosanoic
Cerotic	26	26:0	n-Hexacosanoic
Montanic	28	28:0	n-Octacosanoic

Unsaturated Fatty Acids			
Palmitoleic	16	16:1	Hexadecenoic
Oleic	18	18:1	Octadecenoic
Linoleic	18	18:2	Octadecadienoic
Linolenic	18	18:3	Octadecatrienoic
Arachidonic	20	20:4	Eicosatetraenoic
Erucic	22	22:1	Docosenoic

APPENDIX V

Xenoestrogens/Phytochemicals and Phytoestrogens

Xenoestrogens In The Environment

A recent study found that professional women golfers had a much higher incidence of breast cancer than the general population-possibly attributed to the chemicals used on golf courses. Long Island women in Nassau and Suffolk counties have had excessively high rates of breast cancer-possibly due to the willy-nilly spraying of DDT over residential areas in both counties in the 50's. Women with breast cancer often have unusually high levels of organochlorines (PCB, DDT) in their blood, indicating exposure at some time. Xenoestrogens like DDT and organochlorines are known to enhance the metabolic conversion of the hormone Estradiol to 16-alpha-hydroxyestrone instead of the other, less potent estrogen, 2-alpha-hydroxyestrone. 16HE stimulates division of breast cancer cells more than 2HE does.

Where do these estrogens come from? Just about everywhere. Lawn chemicals are one way you introduce them into your life. Breast cancer is a common result. If you feel like their might be a genetic component to breast cancer, forget it. Firstly, only 5% of all breast cancers are a result of possible genetic links. Secondly, there's virtually nothing you can do to change your inheritance, so focusing on food and environmental causes and cures is the only answer.

Are other species or men affected? Yes. Dropping sperm counts, testicular cancer in humans, undescended testes in Florida panthers, horrendously crossed beaks in bald eagles, very high testicular cancer in dogs who served in Vietnam, unusually small alligator penises, and dozens of other oddities can be blamed on these xenoestrogens.

And don't look to the pharmaceutical industry for the answers; they're part of the problem. Notice the phrasing and wording in the pamphlets and advertising for any "Cancer Awareness Week" or any of the other cancer informational events. Nowhere will you see any mention of chemicals, pesticides, environmental estrogens or any of the other possible causes of these dreaded diseases. There is a reason. It is large chemical companies which often sponsor such events and not only do they make such chemicals (and refuse to discuss any links), but in one case, at least one of these companies makes the chemicals most often used as a cure. The motivation is economic, not altrustic.

How can we prevent these xenoestrogens from harming us? One way to remove airborne toxins is to have houseplants like Pothos in all rooms of your home. Buy cotton shower curtains to avoid polyphenolic volatiles from new plastic curtains. And stay tuned for any and all information about estrogens in your environment.

Xenoestrogens In The Environment**

Atrazine	Weed Killer
Dieldrin	General insecticide
Chlordane	Termite Killer
DDT	General insecticide
DDE	(from DDT)
Endosulfan	General insecticide
Kepone	Roach/Ant bait
Methoxychlor	General insecticide
PCBs	In electrical insulation, old capacitors and transformers
Bisphenol A	In food plastics-leaches into food in hot conditions
Nonyphenol	In food plastics-leaches out at room temperature
Estrogens	Diethylstlbesterol (DES) given to pregnant women
Hydrocarbons	Aromatic hydrocarbons in the air from gasoline, exhaust, etc

***Note: There are many more than this list contains. Many of these compounds have been banned from use, but linger in our environment for one reason or another.*

Diphenols / Phytoestrogens In our Food

Diphenolic compounds like isoflavonoids and lignans are known to have weak estrogenic activity. In many cases this activity, created when we ingest phytoestrogenic rich foods, has blocked our internal forms of estrogen from creating or promoting cancer.

These compounds block angiogenesis, or new blood vessel formation, which occurs in several situations including tumor promotion. After all, the tumor needs nourishment to grow, so it needs to generate its own blood vessels. Other situations where new blood vessel formation occurs are in wound repair, heart attack, and in pregnancy. From this you should be able to begin to see the yin-yang of phytoestrogenic compounds. On the good side, they inhibit the breast and colon cancer gene (the *ras* oncogene) from becoming activated. and they induce apoptosis (destruction) of damaged cells.

Diphenols / Phytoestrogens In our Food

Genistein	Soy, Flax
Diadzein	Soy, Flax
Equol	Soy, Flax
Biochanin A	(Genistein precursor)
Formonetin	(Genistein precursor)
Glycetin	(Genistein precursor)
Coniferyl alcohol	Soy sauce (Lignan precursor)
Ellagic Acid	Strawberries, walnuts

Other Phytochemicals In Our Food

I. Simple Phenolics
Simple phenolic compounds have a number of anticancer duties including:
Detoxifying toxins via the liver (Phase II enzymes)
Preventing nitrosamine-formed cancers
Preventing Arachidonic Acid Metabolism-which is potentially carcinogenic
Reversing liver damage from Aflatoxin B-1
Raising DHS hormone-may prevent breast cancer

Simple Phenolics	Sources
Curcumin	Curry, turmeric
3-ethylphenol	Chocolate (cocoa beans)
3,4-dimethylphenol	Chocolate (cocoa beans)
Capsaicin	Chili pepper
Carnosol	Sage, Rosemary
Coumarin	Vanilla, cloves, nutmeg
p-Cresol	Berries
Eugenol	Cloves
Gallic Acid	Coffee, strawberries
Gingerol	Ginger
Hydroquinone	Sesame seeds
Menthol	Mint
Myristicin	Nutmeg
Piperine	Black pepper
Safrole	Nutmeg, black pepper
Sesamol	Sesame seeds
Shogoal	Ginger
Thymol	Eucalyptus and related genera
Vanillin	Vanilla bean
Zingbain	Ginger

II. Hydroxycinnamic Acid Derivatives
Hydroxycinnamic acid derivatives are linked with a reduction in colon cancer and lipid peroxidation (a precursor to cancer). They also inhibit nitrosamine formation-the compounds formed in your stomach after you eat barbequed meat, for example.

Hydroxycinnamic Acid Derivatives	
Caffeic Acid	Coffee
Chlorogenic Acid	Coffee, berries
Ferulic Acid	Soybeans, berries
p-Coumaric Acid	Soybeans, berries
Quercetin	Coffee, onions, many fruits/veg

III. Flavonoids

High flavonoid intake appears to be preventative of heart disease according to studies in the Netherlands and Finland. Flavonoids reduce clotting and scavenge free radicals. They are also anticarcinogenic; they inhibit activation of a carcinogen, inhibit Arachidonic acid metabolism, and they change proliferation and growth rates of tumors. Flavonoids also modify signal transduction (cell to cell or internal contact) by inhibiting several protein kinase enzymes and polyamine metabolism. They can prevent the changeover from regular cell to cancer cell as well.

Flavonoids	
Anthocyanins	Red wine, red vegetables/fruits
Catechins	Tea, red wine, fruit
Flavonols	Apple, onions, mushrooms

IV. Indoles

Indoles are augmented by plant cell injury, such as cutting or chewing. They help with detoxification of toxins. They stimulate Phase I and Phase II liver detoxification enzyme reactions. They also block the action of creatinine which is suspect in the cancer-causing IQ (Aminoamidazo compounds) formation.

Indoles	
Indole-3-Carbinol (I3C)	Broccoli & Crucifers
Indole(3,2-b) Carbizole (I3Z)	Crucifers (formed in stomach)
Indole-3-Acetonitrile (IAN)	Crucifers
L-tryptophan*	Protein foods
	(*mutagenic if heated)

V. Isothiocyanates

These glucosinolate compounds are released and turned into isothiocyanates when plant cells are damaged and release myrosinase (a conversion enzyme). They can inhibit nitrosamine (NNK, BAP) induced cancers and lung cancer. These isothiocyanates also induce the Phase II liver detoxification enzymes. Sulforaphane was found to inhibit breast cancer this way.

Isothiocyanates	
Phenethyl isothiocyanate (PEITC)	Turnips, crucifers, watercress
Sulforaphane	Broccoli, cabbage
Benzyl isothiocyanate (BITC)	Broccoli, cabbage

VI. Monoterpenes

These are found in essential oils in plants, like mint and rosemary. Orange peel, lemon oil, dill weed, caraway, thyme, cardamom, coriander and celery have lots of limonene. Here, once again, we have the unusual dichotomy which separates oxidized and unoxidized compounds. Fresh, unoxidized limonene can prevent breast, stomach, skin and liver cancer (in rodents), while oxidized limonene causes rampant cancer in other studies. The key is the form in which it's presented to the subject or tissue.

Monoterpenes	
Menthol	Mint
Eucalyptol	Eucalyptus leaves
D-Limonene	Orange peel, etc.
D-Carvone	Caraway, dill
Perryl Alcohol	Cherries

VII. Carotenoids

Carotenoids are fat-soluble compounds which give an orange or yellow color to vegetables and fruits. Lycopene, a tomato carotenoid, is responsible for the red color of ripe tomatoes. All carotenoids are strong antioxidants, and equally strong pro-oxidants as the smokers who took them in the Finnish study found out.

Isolated betacarotene (in the Finnish Betacarotene study) caused and accelerated cancer in those who had smoked for many years and who were using it in this study to show how well it prevented cancer. Whoops! In fact, cancer was up 18% from the control patients in the study. It should be noted that only one isomer (or form) of Betacarotene was used. According to Paul Lachance of The Nutraceutical Institute at Rutgers University, there are 272 different forms of isolated carotene, and only one was used in this study. He feels as though they might have worked synergistically (in a beneficial way) had more of them been present in the 20 mg betacarotene supplement given to the subjects. An interesting note, though, is that many of these unlucky victims of a premise gone wrong were also heavy drinkers. Again, if you don't get it from food, it is liable to be oxidized and could harm you.

Carotenoids	
Betacarotene	Carrots, apricots, tomatoes, peaches
Lutein	Spinach, winter squash, brocolli
Lycopene	Tomatoes, pink grapefruit, apricot
Zeaxanthin	Corn, green peas, mango, kale
Cyrptoxanthin	Oranges, peaches, papaya

APPENDIX VI

Herbal/Organic Information

Herbal / Organic Information

Informational Sources
Alternative Medicine
www.althealthsearch.com
www.healthexplorer.com
www.altmedicine.com
www.aubrey-organics.com

American Botanical Council
www.herbalgram.org
(800) 373-7105 for publications

Natural Heartburn Remedies
Stop The Heartburn
Dr. David Utley (1996)

National Cancer Institute
www.icic.nci.nih.com

Council Against Health Fraud
www.primenet.com

U.S. Department Of Agriculture
www.usda.gov

Vegetarian Resource Group
www.envirolink.org/arrs/vrg/home/
html

Vegetarian Times
www.vegetariantimes.com

Responsible Or Organic Food Companies
Eden Organic Foods
(800) 248-0230
(888) 2124-EDEN

Amy's Kitchen, Inc.
P.O. Box 449
Petaluma, CA 94543
(707)762-6194

Celestial Seasonings
4600 Sleepytime Drive
Boulder, CO 80301-3292

Lightlife Foods, Inc.
P.O. Box 870
Greenfield, MA 01302
(800) 274-6001

Juniper Valley Organic Milk
P.O. Box 278 Route 30
Roxbury, NY 12474

Ben & Jerry's Ice Cream
30 Community Drive
South Burlington, VT 05403-6828
(802) 651-9600

Nest Eggs, Inc.
P.O. Box 14599
Chicago, IL 60614
(773) 525-4952

Vegetarian Pets
Wow-Bow Distributors Ltd.
13 B Lucon Drive
Deer Park, NY 11729
(800)-326-0230

PetSage
www.petsage.com
(800) PET-HLTH

Alternative Medications

As with all advice in this guide, these medications are not offered here as prescriptive, but rather as the typical dosages and types of medications that are popular in the alternative market. Do not substitute any of these herbal preparations or alternatives for prescribed drugs. Do not take these with prescription drugs without checking with your doctor or pharmacist first.

Ailment: Aches & Pains
OTC Preparation: Aspirin / Tylenol
Alternatives: Omega-3 (In Fish; Flax) (2 gm/d); Feverfew (In Tea) (400 ug/d); Natural salicylates (In Tea); Magnesium (Green Veg.) (300 mg/d); Pycnogenol (Cranberries) (50 mg/d); Capsaicin (Hot peppers) (4x/d); Garlic (any form) (600mg/d)

Ailment: Colds
OTC Preparation: Nyquil / Tylenol
Alternatives: Zinc lozenges (3/d); Vitamin C (In fruit) (1g/d); Vitamin E (In nuts, oils) (60mg/d); Beta-carotene (see Vit.A) (10mg/d); Ma Huang (Ephedra tea); Echinacea tea (500 mg/d); Garlic (any form) (600 mg/d)

Ailment: Stomach Upset
OTC Preparation: Pepto Bismol, Tagamet, Rolaids, Pepcid AC, Zantac
Alternatives: Licorice root tea (1.4 g/d); Probiotic (Yogurt) (1,8 oz/d); Probiotic (Kefir); Plain Water (8 -16 oz/d); Peppermint tea (2 c/d); Green Tea (2 c/d)

Ailment: Infection
OTC Preparation: Penicillin, Biaxin, Amoxicillin, Cephlex
Alternatives: Garlic (any form) (600mg/d); Alcohol (12%) (1 glass/d); Yogurt (1,8oz/d); Echinacea (500mg/d); Grapefruit (2halves/d)

Ailment: Constipation
OTC Preparation: X-Lax, Metamucil, Mineral Oil
Alternatives: Exercise (20min/d); Bran Cereal (1cup/d); Prunes (2-3/d); Plain Water (16+oz/d); High Fiber (5 Fruits)

Ailment: Heart Trouble
OTC Preparation: Vasotec
Alternatives: Aspirin (81mg/d); Magnesium (300mg/d); Garlic (600mg/d); Calcium (1g/d); Bananas (2/day).

APPENDIX VII

Food Allergy

Food Allergy

Food Allergy Or Food Intolerance?

Imagine being kissed by someone who just ate a peanut and dying from the encounter? It has happened. It is not that unusual for a whiff of shrimp passing to the next table at a restaurant or minute amounts of almond extract in a tiny forkful of dessert to create an immediate life-threatening situation for those hypersensitive to food ingredients.

Both food allergies and food intolerances can be very serious and should be diagnosed by a Board certified allergist (an M.D.). This is a medical issue, not a nutritional one. Do not trust your life or your child's life to anyone who claims to be a good diagnoser of allergies, a nutritionist, a clinical ecologist, or anyone who is not an M.D. Below are some guidelines for telling what you might have. These guidelines will be useful to understand what your physician will tell you. Do not use these to diagnose yourself. Only a qualified physician can make your diagnosis.

The 8 Types of Food That Causes 90+% of All Food Allergies	
Food	**Possible Allergen**
Milk	Casein, Lactoglobulin, Lactalbumin
Egg	
White	Ovomucoid, Ovalbumin, Conalbumin
Yolk	Lipoprotein, Apovitellenin, Livetin
Wheat	Albumin, Globulin
Crustacea	Parvalbumin, Antigen I
Mollusks	Antigen I, Antigen II, Parvalbumin
Fish	Allergen M
Legumes	Glycinin, Kunitz Trypsin Inhibitor, Concanavalin
Tree Nuts	Several unidentified proteins

Which Foods Contain These Allergens?

Milk
Milk, yogurt, cheese, ice cream, any dairy product
Egg
All bird eggs, baked goods, noodles
Wheat
Bread, cereal, pasta
Crustaceans
Shrimp, crab, lobster, crayfish
Mollusks
Clams, oysters, scallops, etc.
Fish
Cod, haddock, salmon, etc.
Legumes
Green peas, peanuts, soybeans

Typical Allergic Symptoms And Location

Skin
Rash, hives, eczema

Mouth
Tongue or lips swell or itch

Trachea/ Bronchii
Breathing difficulties, rhinitis, runny nose

Digestive Tract
Vomiting, diarrhea, pains

It's Probably Not Food Allergy If You
Have a delayed reaction

GI problems, but no Immune response

Cannot digest milk (Lactase deficiency)
Cannot digest sugars (Sucrase deficiency)
Cannot digest Phenylalanine (Phenylketonuria)

React to Bacterial toxins (Botulinum or Staph)
React to Fungal toxins (Aflatoxin, Ergot)
React to Fish toxins (Saxitoxin, Domoic acid, Ciguatoxin)

React to typical food chemicals like:
Tyramine (If on MAO inhibitors; in cheese, herring, wine)
Histamine (Scombroid poisoning)
Caffeine (Coffee, tea)
Alcohol (All)
Theobromine (In chocolate, tea)
Tartrazine (Yellow #5)
Nitrates (Ham, sausage, jerky)
Sulfites (Dried fruit, wine)
MSG (Chinese food, prepared soups) |

It's Probably A Food Allergy If

There is an immediate reaction

There is an immune response
(IgE released)

Reaction follows consumption of or exposure to one of the major
allergens listed above (The 8 Major Allergens)

The patient is a child. More food allergies occur in children than adults.
Only 1-2% of the adult population has food allergies. The number is 3-
4% for children.

APPENDIX VIII

U.S. Food Festivals

U.S. Food Festivals
(most are Pet-Friendly!)

Apple Harvest Festival (October) Southington, CT
(860) 225-3901
French Festival of NewEngland(June) Newport, RI
(401) 683-1479
Strawberry Wine Festival LinganoreWine Cellars, MD
(301) 831-5889
Blueberry Wine Festival LinganoreWine Cellars, MD
(301) 831-5889
Reggae Festival LinganoreWine Cellars, MD
(301) 831-5889
Bayou Razz-Jazz Festival LinganoreWine Cellars, MD
(301) 831-5889
Strawberry Festival (Summer) Chester, NJ
(908) 879-5541
Peach Festival (Summer) Chester, NJ
(908) 879-5541
Apple Festival (Fall) Chester, NJ
(908) 879-5541
Upper Ohio Valley Italian Festival (July) Wheeling, WV
(304) 828-3097
World's Largest Peanut Boil (Summer) Luverne, AL
(334) 335-5516
Sand Mountain Potato Festival (June) Henager, AL
(205) 657-5849
Jay Grelen's Sweet Tea Sip-Off (Summer) Mobile, AL
(334) 973-2217
Wine Festival (October) Santa Rosa Beach, FL
(904) 267-8092

Oktoberfest (October) Savannah, GA
(912) 234-0295
Biloxi Seafood Fest (Summer)Biloxi, MS
(800) 237-9493
Berghoff Oktoberfest (September) Chicago, IL
(312) 427-3170
A Taste Of Chicago (June) Chicago, IL
(312) 744-3315
Popcorn Festival (September) Valparaiso, IN
(800) 283-8687
International Banana Festival (September) Fulton, KY
(502) 472-2975
Kentucky Bourbon Festival (September) Bardstown, KY
(502) 349-0804
Mushroom Festival (May) Mesick, MI
(616) 885-1280
Pasty Bake (May) St. Ignace, MI
(800) 338-6660
Cereal Festival (June) Battle Creek, MI
(616) 962-8400
Zuccini Festival (Summer) Eldorado, OH
(513) 273-3281
Food, Folks and Spokes (July) Kenosha, WI
(414) 657-5031
Picklefest (July) Atkins, AR
(501) 641-2576
French Quarter Festival (April) New Orleans, LA
(504) 522-5730
Ardmore Birthday Party (May) Ardmore, OK
(405) 223-7765
Pecan Festival (June) Okmulgee, OK
(918) 756-6172

Chili Festival (October) Okmulgee, OK
(918) 756-6172
Annual Sweet Onion Festival (June) Rock Springs, AZ
(602) 465-9256
Dry Bean Festival (August) Tracy, CA
(209) 835-2131
Nisei Week Japanese Festival (August) Los Angeles, CA
(213) 687-7193
Monterey Wine Makers Festival (August) Monterey, CA
(408) 375-9400
Oktoberfest (October) Denver,CO
(303) 534-2367
Bat Flight Breakfast (August) Carlsbad, NM
(800) 221-1224
Hatch Chili Festival Hatch, NM
(505) 267-5050
Henry Goes Wines Umpqua, OR
(541) 459-5120

References / Suggested Reading

Animals Without Backbones, Buchsbaum, R. et. al., University of Chicago Press, 1987.

"Antimutagens as chemopreventive agents in the diet" Ferguson, L., Mutation Research 307 (1994) Elsevier Science Publishers

Basic Microbiology, Volk, W.A., Harper Collins, 1992.

Basic Medical Microbiology, Boyd, R.F. et. al., Little, Brown and Company, 1996.

Biology of Microorganisms, Brock, T.D., Prentice-Hall, 1988.

"Characterization of the influences of organic, low-input, and conventional growing practices on attributes of Lycopersicon esculentum" Walters, H.M., Rutgers University, 1995.

Contemporary Nutrition, Wardlaw, G.M. et. al., 1994/1997, Mosby Publishers.

Deadly Feasts, Rhodes, R., Simon & Schuster, 1997.

The Drinking Water Book, Ingram, C., Ten Speed Press, 1995.

Dr. Susan Love's Hormone Book, Love, S., Random House, 1997.

Estrogen: The Natural Way, Shandler, N., Villard, 1997.

Food Chemistry, Fennema, O.R., 1985/1996, Marcel Dekker, Inc.

Fundamentals of Microanalytical Entomology, Olsen, A.R. et. al., CRC Press, 1996.

Human Biology, Chiras, D., West Publishing Company, 1991.

"Inhibitory effect of carnosolic acid on HIV-1 protease in cell-free assays", Paris, A. et. al., Journal of Natural Products 1993.

Natural Woman, Natural Menopause, Conrad, C., Harper-Collins, 1997.

"Nutritional responsibilities of food companies in the next century", Lachance, P., Food Technology, 1989.

Nutrition, Nieman et. al., Wm. C. Brown Publishers, 1990.

Pigments in Vegetables, Gross, J., Van Nostrand Reinhold, 1991.

Plant Vitamins, Mozafar, A., CRC Press, 1994.

"Potential Dangers of Iron Overload in Rich American Diet", Brody, J., The New York Times, 1997.

Prevention, Rodale Press, Emmaus, PA (610) 967-5171.

"Progress in the identification of irradiated foods", Stevenson, M.H., Trends in Food Science & Technology, 1992.

"Regular Exercise Protects Women Against Breast Cancer", Gina Colada, The New York Times, 1997.

Sensory Evaluation Techniques, 2nd Edition, Meilgaard, Civille, and Carr, CRC Press, 1991.

"Soy component genistein may protect against breast cancer", Barnes, S., Food Chemistry News, 1994.

Index

About The Author

Dr. Heather MacLean Walters has taught many undergraduate and graduate level courses. She has lectured for community groups, schools and professional associations like The New Jersey Dietetic Association.   Courses she has taught include Advanced Medical Nutrition, Nutrition, Nutritional Biochemistry, Chemistry, Organic Chemistry, Biology, Microbiology, and Organismal Genetics. She has her undergraduate degree in Molecular Biology from Cornell University, a Masters in Environmental Biology from University of Massachusetts, a Masters in Biology Curriculum from the University of Massachusetts, and a PhD in Food Biology from Rutgers University.

Dr. Walters' desire is to inform, educate, and incite change of programs and services that aren't working to help protect our food system. But *you* are the agents of change. *You* must bring your knowledge to the proper individuals and ask them to fix what is broken, to leave alone that which is good and to support programs to insure your safety. She cannot do this alone. She needs your help.